"Adam B. Lewin and Eric A. Storch, two of the world's experts, have assembled a highly insightful and practical volume to help those with any level of experience better understand and treat children with OCD. This book is a must for any student or professional working in the field."

—*Jonathan S. Abramowitz, Professor of Psychology and Director of the OCD Program at University of North Carolina at Chapel Hill*

"A wonderfully accessible read, full of down-to-earth information but thoroughly up to date. Written by a team of recognized experts in the field in a way that allows the medical and non-medical reader to fully grasp all aspects of this disorder and negotiate treatment decisions for themselves, their loved ones, and their patients with confidence. A valuable book for consumers and professionals alike."

—*Daniel Geller, MD, Director of the Pediatric OCD and Tic Disorder Program and Michele and David Mittelman Family Chair of Child and Adolescent Psychiatry at Massachusetts General Hospital, Associate Professor of Psychiatry at Harvard Medical School*

"Doctors Lewin and Storch have crafted a reader-friendly, insightful text that will be useful for any provider hoping to learn more about OCD, or any parent who has a child struggling with OCD. Doctors Lewin and Storch should be congratulated for this masterful work, which fills a critical gap in the field of childhood OCD."

—*Wayne Goodman, MD, Professor and Chair, Menninger Department of Psychiatry and Behavioral Sciences, Baylor College of Medicine, Texas*

"This is one of the most complete and warm-hearted books I have read about people who fight to deal with intrusive thoughts. Readers are given detailed information of what it means to have unwanted intrusive thoughts, as well as the origin and impact of these thoughts on the emotional and social life of people diagnosed with OCD. The book provides both practical and research-based guidance to readers and is a must-read for anyone experiencing such thoughts, as well as the people who are involved in their lives (family, friends, and professionals)."

—*Ioannis Voskopoulos, Psychologist at TNA*

of related interest

Can I Tell you about OCD?
A guide for friends, family and professionals
Amita Jassi
Illustrated by Sarah Hull
ISBN 978 1 84905 381 5
eISBN 978 0 85700 736 0
Can I tell you about...?

Breaking Free from OCD
A CBT Guide for Young People and Their Families
Jo Derisley, Isobel Heyman, Sarah Robinson and Cynthia Turner
ISBN 978 1 84310 574 9
eISBN 978 1 84642 799 2

Parenting OCD
Down to Earth Advice From One Parent to Another
Claire Sanders
ISBN 978 1 84905 478 2
eISBN 978 0 85700 916 6

UNDERSTANDING
OCD

A GUIDE FOR PARENTS AND PROFESSIONALS

Edited by Adam B. Lewin
and Eric A. Storch

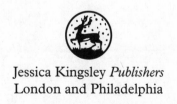

Jessica Kingsley *Publishers*
London and Philadelphia

First published in 2017
by Jessica Kingsley Publishers
73 Collier Street
London N1 9BE, UK
and
400 Market Street, Suite 400
Philadelphia, PA 19106, USA

www.jkp.com

Library of Congress Cataloging in Publication Data
Title: Understanding OCD : a guide for parents and professionals / edited by
    Adam Lewin and Eric Storch.
Other titles: Understanding obsessive-compulsive disorder
Description: London ; Philadelphia : Jessica Kingsley Publishers, 2017. |
    Includes bibliographical references and index.
Identifiers: LCCN 2016046952 (print) | LCCN 2016047837 (ebook) | ISBN
    9781849057837 (alk. paper) | ISBN 9781784500269 (ebook)
Subjects: LCSH: Obsessive-compulsive disorder--Treatment. |
    Obsessive-compulsive disorder--Diagnosis.
Classification: LCC RC533 .U54 2017 (print) | LCC RC533 (ebook) | DDC
    616.85/227--dc23

British Library Cataloguing in Publication Data
A CIP catalogue record for this book is available from the British Library

ISBN 978 1 84905 783 7
eISBN 978 1 78450 026 9

Printed and bound in the United States

In memory of HG.

ADAM B. LEWIN

With love to EMS, NRS, MLS, and JFS. And, to the many families who have given me the honor of working with and learning from them.

ERIC A. STORCH

Contents

INTRODUCTION

Eric A. Storch and Adam B. Lewin

Pediatric obsessive compulsive disorder (OCD) is a common condition that affects about 1 to 2 percent of children and adolescents. It causes considerable problems for children and their loved ones in most areas of life. Parents and other family members of a child with OCD often feel helpless with how to help their loved one effectively deal with OCD. Over the past several decades, however, clinicians and researchers have learned much more about OCD among children, and, most importantly, how to address it. More specifically, two types of effective treatments have been established. These include a form of psychotherapy called cognitive behavioral therapy (CBT) with exposure and response prevention (ERP) as well as a group of medicines called serotonin reuptake inhibitors (SRIs). This book speaks primarily of how to understand childhood OCD, and the potential role of CBT in helping to address it.

In our collective 30 years of experience working with individuals with OCD, one of the things we have noticed in working with families of a child affected with OCD is that family members have many questions about the nature of

OCD and how CBT works. Good providers are usually able to explain most of these, but sometimes something may not make sense, or one may want to have a book to give a loved one who cannot make it to sessions. We have also noticed that not all providers know about how to provide effective CBT, and we wanted to create a resource that gives additional information about this treatment. Yet, there was not a readily available source that described childhood OCD or explained the components of CBT in a manner that would be easily understood and—most importantly— easy to read for parents, family members, and providers who are interested in learning more. Because of this we decided to recruit experts in childhood OCD to provide descriptions of the core components of CBT treatment as well as features related to OCD.

This book is divided into three parts consisting of several practical, easy to read but also not simplified chapters appreciating the considerable expertise that many parents develop in trying to help their child with OCD. We recruited leading researchers and clinicians to contribute their perspective on the subject matter. The first part provides an overview of childhood OCD. The second part discusses CBT for children with OCD and their families. Finally, the third part discusses an array of issues common to OCD such as ensuring the right level of care, how to address OCD at school and at home, and things that might relate to a child being successful in treatment.

The first chapter in Part 1 starts by describing the nature of childhood OCD including the types of symptoms that commonly occur as well as problems that often co-occur such as anxiety and depression. Next, there are two chapters that discuss theories related to how OCD is caused and why symptoms last. A chapter is then included teaching parents and those who work with children how to recognize OCD in youth. The final chapter of Part 1 summarizes current research on the treatment of childhood OCD and how to decide on the best approach for a particular child. Part 2 has five chapters. The first is an overview of CBT for childhood OCD with a focus on education about the disorder and its treatment. Next, a chapter discussing key CBT approaches including building a fear hierarchy, ERP, and challenging obsessive compulsive and anxious thoughts. The following chapter discusses how to choose the right level of care based on the problems the child is presenting with. The final two chapters discuss information about factors that are related to outcome as well as how to maximize improvements, and discusses what to do when treatments does not work. Part 3 includes two chapters discussing OCD at school and at home. The chapter on OCD at school provides an overview for parents and educators about how OCD affects education and strategies for overcoming it within a school setting. The chapter on OCD at home discusses helping parents manage their child's OCD in the home setting.

It is our hope that this book makes a meaningful contribution by spreading knowledge about OCD during childhood as well as how to effectively treat it with CBT. We believe that this book could serve as a companion for the loved ones of someone who is receiving CBT to complement the therapeutic work that is being done as well as to provide insight into the therapy components and techniques. It is also our hope that this book will provide therapists with a resource at their disposal to learn more about this intervention given how well it works and the great need to improve its availability.

PART 1

Overview of Childhood Obsessive Compulsive Disorder

1

WHAT IS OBSESSIVE COMPULSIVE DISORDER?

Caleb W. Lack[1]

Whether a person is a parent or a professional who is new to obsessive compulsive disorder (OCD), one of the first questions I often hear is "What exactly is OCD?" For many people, if they are familiar with OCD at all it is primarily through portrayals in the media. From the brilliant but impaired detective on *Monk* to the lead character from HBO's *Girls* to the hilarious Bill Murray in *What About Bob?* there is no shortage of television or movie characters that purport to have OCD. You may have also heard the term used in everyday language by people saying things like "Oh, I'm a little OCD" about cleaning or germs or some other thing. The purpose of this chapter is to help you get a better, scientifically informed understanding about what OCD is and is not. As you will learn, what people think they know about OCD and what OCD actually is are often two quite different things.

1 Correspondence concerning this chapter should be addressed to Caleb W. Lack, Ph.D., Department of Psychology, College of Education and Professional Studies, University of Central Oklahoma, 100 North University Drive, Edmond, OK 73034. E-mail: clack@uco.edu.

Diagnostically, OCD is a mental disorder that is primarily diagnosed based upon the presence of *obsessions* and/or *compulsions* (APA 2013). The *Diagnostic and Statistical Manual of Mental Disorders, Fifth Edition* (DSM-5; the most current version of the "bible" of mental health diagnoses) defines obsessions as unwelcome and distressing ideas, thoughts, images or impulses that repetitively occur; and compulsions as behaviors or actions that an individual feels a need to perform and are often difficult to resist. Far from being odd or unusual experiences, most people have experienced non-clinical levels of obsessions and compulsions at some point in their lives (Abramowitz *et al.* 2014). Obsessing over an upcoming event (e.g., an exam or interview); worrying that you forgot to lock the front door or turn off the stove before leaving for a trip; always having your desk organized in a specific way; performing superstitious behaviors (e.g., always wearing a particular sports jersey on days that your favorite team plays): these are all examples of some minor obsessions and compulsions. Insignificant obsessions and compulsions are harmless and can actually prove to be beneficial to individuals. Ritualistic behaviors (or compulsions), such as taking time to organize one's desk at the start or end of a workday can create a sense of relief and reduce anxiety. This may be why routines and rituals are extremely common among children and adults, from sleeping in the same position every night to buttoning your shirt in a particular fashion (Kanner 2005).

In other words, almost all of us are "a little bit OCD," but only if by that you mean that you have some obsessive thoughts or compulsive behaviors from time to time. As with most other aspects of human life, obsessions and compulsions exist on a continuum, from the minor ones most people have to majorly impairing ones that will result in a diagnosis of OCD. Much like many other thoughts and behaviors, obsessions and compulsions only become problematic when they are carried out excessively, irrationally, for unreasonable amounts of time, to a level that causes significant distress to the person, or when they hinder daily living (Lack 2013).

The diagnosis of OCD

OCD is not in any way a "new" disorder. In fact, references to symptoms of what we now call obsessive compulsive disorder date back hundreds of years. Case studies and reports from history make it clear that OCD has been with the human species for a very long time, from Lady Macbeth's excessive hand washing to Martin Luther's excessive scrupulosity (Krochmalik and Menzies 2003). Attempts to really understand OCD began in the early 1800s, and it was viewed as "insanity with insight" because persons suffering from OCD did not have the disconnect from reality seen in psychosis (what we would today call schizophrenia; Salzman and Thaler 1981). A more contemporary understanding began by the early twentieth century, with several psychological frameworks for understanding why people had OCD competing for attention. Today, it is generally accepted that people who have OCD do so because of a combination of biological, psychological, and social factors, rather than just "one thing" causing it (Lack *et al.* 2015).

Concurrent with an increasing understanding of OCD was the development of diagnostic criteria. As diagnostic guidelines for mental disorders were developed in the twentieth century, two systems rose to prominence. The *Diagnostic and Statistical Manual for Mental Disorders*

(DSM), published by the American Psychiatric Association, is currently the most widely used manual by mental health clinicians to define the symptoms of what are variously called mental disorders, mental illness, or psychopathology (including OCD) in the United States. The next most popular diagnostic manual that clinicians use, both outside and inside the US, is the *International Statistical Classification of Diseases and Related Health Problems* (ICD), currently in its tenth revision. Below we will cover how these guidelines are similar and different.

The DSM is currently on its fifth revision and contains some major changes in how OCD is conceptualized compared to prior versions. In the DSM-IV (APA 2000), OCD was classified as an anxiety disorder (as it was in all prior versions) while in the DSM-5 it has been removed from the anxiety disorders and placed in a new section titled "Obsessive-Compulsive and Related Disorders." The other disorders in this section are body dysmorphic disorder, trichotillomania or hair-pulling, hoarding, and excoriation or skin-picking. The DSM-5 notes, however, that the "Obsessive-Compulsive and Related Disorders" section was purposefully placed right after the "Anxiety Disorders" section because of the shared characteristics between anxiety and obsessive-compulsive symptoms. Even with that consideration, it was and remains a highly controversial decision to remove OCD from the "Anxiety Disorders" and create a new category that it apparently exemplifies.

A section change was not the only OCD-related change given consideration when the DSM-5 was being developed. Changing of the wording in the diagnostic criteria for OCD was also debated, but only some small changes were made. For example, in item 1 under Obsessions the word "impulses" (DSM-IV-TR) was changed to "urges" (DSM-5). While "impulse" and "urge" both represent the seemingly uncontrollable drive associated with obsessions, "impulse" may confuse or influence clinicians and lead them to make an inaccurate diagnosis by confusing it with the impulse control disorders (Leckman *et al.* 2010). Other wording changes were also made, but do not significantly impact the diagnosis. Given these small changes, only the diagnostic criteria from the DSM-5 will be discussed.

The first criterion that must be met for a diagnosis of OCD is experiencing obsessions, compulsions, or a combination of the two (which is the most common form). Obsessions are intrusive, unwanted thoughts or urges that cause someone to feel anxious or upset. The person then performs some sort of compulsion in order to try to get those thoughts to go away, so that their anxiety will decrease. Compulsions typically involve repetitive acts that can be either observable behaviors (like hand washing) or mentally performed (like praying or counting). They tend to be very rigidly done (for example, washing one's hands in a very complicated manner for a certain period of time) and happen in response to an obsessive thought. They do not, though, tend to either be realistically related to a feared outcome or, if they are, are obviously excessive in nature.

Next, the person's obsessions and compulsions have to either take a significant amount of time each day or cause impairment in functioning. This often equates to at least one hour per day spent having obsessions or performing compulsive rituals, or someone experiencing problems in being able to interact with family and friends or succeed in school. Further diagnostic criteria are focused on ensuring that a medical condition, substance abuse, or other mental health diagnosis does not better account for what seem to be the OCD symptoms. Finally, the DSM-5 specifies the level of insight an individual has into their symptoms. Someone with good or fair insight is able to tell that their OCD-based beliefs are not likely true, while someone with poor insight thinks that such beliefs are more than likely accurate. A person with absent insight, on the other hand, is totally certain that their OCD-based beliefs are accurate and real.

In the World Health Organization's (WHO) ICD-10, OCD is located in the "Neurotic, Stress-related and Somatoform Disorders" section, which is also where anxiety disorders are. Interestingly, OCD is actually separated from anxiety disorders and given its own subheading (WHO 2010), consistent with its separation in DSM-5. However, they are closely grouped in the ICD-10 and it would be easy to miss this distinction. Another noticeable difference between the DSM-5 and ICD-10 is in the definitions of obsessions and compulsions.

In ICD-10, obsessions are described as:

> ideas, images, or impulses that enter the patient's mind again and again in a stereotyped form. They are almost invariably distressing and the patient often tries, unsuccessfully, to resist them. They are, however, recognized as his or her own thoughts, even though they are involuntary and often repugnant. (WHO 2010, F42.1, p.118)

Compulsions are described as:

> stereotyped behaviours that are repeated again and again. They are not inherently enjoyable, nor do they result in the completion of inherently useful tasks. Their function is to prevent some objectively unlikely event, often involving harm to or caused by the patient, which he or

she fears might otherwise occur. Usually, this behaviour is recognized by the patient as pointless or ineffectual and repeated attempts are made to resist. Anxiety is almost invariably present. If compulsive acts are resisted the anxiety gets worse. (WHO 2010, F42.1, p.118)

Although the wording is a bit different, the basic concepts of what obsessions and compulsions are remains similar. The ICD-10 also specifically notes that obsessions and compulsions are not enjoyable for the individual experiencing them just as the DSM-5 mentions that obsessions are "intrusive and unwanted" (APA 2013).

In contrast to the ICD-10, the DSM-5 directly declares that there is an interactional relationship between obsessions and compulsions (the idea which underlies our most effective treatment, cognitive behavioral therapy—CBT—focusing on exposure and response prevention—ERP). In other words, obsessions are anxiety provoking and compulsions are performed to decrease stress and avoid an imagined unpleasant outcome (e.g., house burning down from leaving the stove on). Although the relief is typically brief in duration, the individual engages in one or more compulsions to alleviate their anxiety. The ICD-10 proclaims that "Underlying the overt behaviour is a fear, usually of danger either to or caused by the patient, and the ritual is an ineffectual or symbolic attempt to avert that danger" (WHO 2010, F42.1, p.118). This references obsessions but does not refer to them directly, which can be a bit confusing for many new to OCD.

Common types of obsessions and compulsions

Contrary to what some may think, the content and purpose of obsessions and compulsions (O/C) seems to differ little between clinical and non-clinical samples (Garcia-Soriano *et al.* 2011). Research has found that while compulsions are not as likely to be overt in non-clinical populations, people without OCD nonetheless engage in anxiety-reducing or anxiety-neutralizing behaviors (i.e., compulsions) when they have obsessive thoughts (Berman *et al.* 2010). Even the most commonly reported O/C, outlined below, are similar between those with and without OCD (Abramowitz *et al.* 2014).

Obsessions can be impulses (a desire to loudly cuss during a funeral), wishes (wishing someone to die), images (imagining your house setting on fire because the oven was left on), or doubts (thinking that you forgot to lock a door) that repeatedly come to mind at a level beyond what would be considered typical worrying over genuine life problems (Challis, Pelling, and Lack 2008). Most often, individuals with obsessions know that the intrusive thoughts are not "normal," which only increases their anxiety. As Table 1.1 shows, obsessions may focus on a variety of themes, including contamination (germs and sickness), aggression and violence (either towards others or self-harm), sexuality, orderliness, religiosity, and extreme uncertainty (fear of forgetting to lock the door or make sure the oven is off before leaving home).

Table 1.1 Most common obsessions seen in OCD

Type of obsession	Examples
Contamination	Bodily fluids, disease, germs, dirt, chemicals, environmental contaminants
Religious obsessions	Blasphemy or offending God, high concern about morality and what is right and wrong
Superstitious ideas	Lucky numbers, colors, words
Perfectionism	Evenness and exactness, "needing" to know or remember, fear of forgetting or losing something
Harm	Fear of hurting others through carelessness, fear of being responsible for something terrible happening
Losing control	Fear of acting on an impulse to harm self or others, fear or unpleasant mental images, fear of saying offending things to others
Unwanted sexual thoughts	Forbidden or "perverse" sexual thoughts, images, or impulses; obsessive thoughts about homosexuality; obsessions involving children or incest; obsessions about aggressive sexual behavior

Compulsions, on the other hand, are repeated actions that are often performed as a means to reduce the anxiety and distress caused by an obsession (Challis, Pelling, and Lack 2008). Obsessions almost always make persons with OCD highly anxious or distressed. Engaging in compulsions can serve to reduce the anxiety caused by obsessions, or sometimes to prevent the anxiety before it occurs; however, the anxiety reduction does not last for very long. While compulsions are performed voluntarily, it does not feel that way to people with OCD. Instead, they believe that something bad will happen if they do not engage in a compulsion (e.g., a loved one will die or they will catch a terrible disease). Compulsive behaviors may be performed anywhere from a few times a day to several hundred times a day, depending on the severity of one's OCD (Abramowitz, Taylor, and McKay 2009). Table 1.2 shows the most common compulsions seen in OCD.

Table 1.2 Most common compulsions seen in OCD

Type of compulsion	Examples
Checking	Making sure that you did not (or will not) harm yourself or others, or that you did not make a mistake, or that nothing "terrible" happened
Repeating	Repeating things in multiples or a certain number of times, certain body movements, rereading or rewriting
Washing/cleaning	Washing hands excessively, excessive showering or bathing, cleaning outside the norm
Mental compulsions	Cancelling out bad thoughts with good ones, counting while walking or performing some task, prayer to prevent something terrible from happening
Hoarding	Collecting items due to compulsions
Ordering and arranging	Putting things in "proper" order or until it "feels right"

As can be seen by comparing the two tables, certain types of obsessions tend to be "paired up" with certain types of compulsions. For example, contamination obsessions are most often followed by washing or cleaning compulsions to help neutralize them. Religious obsessions are typically paired with mental compulsions of prayer. Understanding these typical patterns can help when working with individuals who do not have much insight into their own mind and behavior, as you can often infer which obsession is present based on the compulsion and then use that inference to guide questions and assessment.

Epidemiological aspects of OCD

In the US, the lifetime prevalence rate of OCD is estimated at 2.3 percent in adults (Kessler *et al.* 2005) and around 1–2.3 percent in children and adolescents under 18 (Zohar 1999). There are also about 5 percent of the population who are "sub-clinical" cases of OCD, experiencing some impairment but not meeting full diagnostic criteria (Ruscio *et al.* 2010). There is strong evidence that cultural differences do not play a prominent role in presence of OCD, with research showing few epidemiological differences across different countries. There are, however, cultural influences on symptom expression (see Williams and Steever 2015 for a thorough review).

While OCD is equally present in males and females in adulthood, the disorder is heavily male in pediatric patients (Geller 2006). There are some differences in comorbidity as well. Among men, hoarding symptoms are most often associated with generalized anxiety disorder (GAD) and tic disorders, but in women social anxiety, post-traumatic stress disorder (PTSD), body dysmorphic disorder, nail-biting, and skin-picking are more often observed (Kessler *et al.* 2005; Torres *et al.* 2006).

Presentation of OCD symptoms is generally the same in children and adults (Stewart *et al.* 2008). Unlike many adults, though, younger children will not be able to recognize that their obsessions and compulsions are both unnecessary (e.g., you don't really need to wash your hands) and extreme (e.g., washing hands for 15–20 seconds is fine, but five minutes in scalding water is too much). In young children, compulsions often occur without the patient being able to report their obsessions, while adolescents are often able to report multiple obsessions and compulsions. Children and adolescents are also more likely to include family members in their rituals and can be highly demanding of adherence to rituals and rules, leading to disruptive and oppositional behavior. As such, youth with OCD are generally more impaired than adults with the same type of symptoms (Piacentini *et al.* 2007).

Up to 75 percent of persons with OCD qualify for other mental health diagnoses (Kessler 2005). The most common in pediatric cases are attention deficit hyperactivity disorder (ADHD), disruptive behavior disorders, major depression, and other anxiety disorders (Geller *et al.* 1996). In adults, the most prevalent comorbids are social anxiety, major depression, and alcohol abuse (Torres *et al.* 2006). Interestingly, the presence of comorbid diagnoses predicts quality of life more so than OCD severity itself in both children and adults (Fontenelle *et al.* 2010; Lack *et al.* 2009). Different primary O/C are also associated with certain patterns of comorbidity, in both adults and youth. Primary symmetry/ordering symptoms are often seen with comorbid tics, bipolar disorder, obsessive compulsive personality disorder, panic disorder, and agoraphobia, while those with contamination/cleaning symptoms are more likely to be diagnosed with an eating disorder. Those with hoarding cluster symptoms, on the other hand, are especially likely to be diagnosed with personality disorders, particularly Cluster C disorders (De Mathis *et al.* 2006).

Impairment issues related to OCD

Almost all individuals with OCD experience both obsessions and compulsions (APA 2013). As such, people with OCD spend a large amount of time (usually more than one hour per day) performing their compulsions and thinking obsessively (Challis *et al.* 2008). The O/C make even the easiest of daily chores or activities time consuming and stressful, with almost all adults and children with OCD reporting that their obsessions cause them significant distress and anxiety, as opposed to similar, intrusive thoughts in persons without OCD (Subramaniam *et al.* 2013).

In terms of quality of life (QoL), persons with OCD report a pervasive decrease compared to those without OCD. Youth show problematic peer relations, academic difficulties, and participate in fewer recreational activities than matched peers (Lack *et al.* 2009). Overall, there is a lower QoL in pediatric females than males, but in adults similar disruptions are reported. When compared to anxiety disorders and depressive disorders, a person with OCD is less likely to be married, more likely to be unemployed, and more likely to report impaired social and occupational functioning (Macy *et al.* 2013).

Daily, there are a number of problems that people with OCD face. One example is the avoidance of situations in which the objects of the obsessions are present. For example, a person may avoid using public restrooms or shaking hands with people because doing so will trigger their contamination obsession, which will lead to them having to do a cleansing compulsion. One middle-aged male that I saw for treatment had avoided taking a shower for several months at the time of our first meeting, because the compulsions he had to perform while cleaning himself resulted in showers lasting five or more hours at a time. Some people will not leave their homes because that is the only way to avoid objects and situations that will trigger their obsessions. Frequent doctor visits may also occur because they fear that something is wrong with them physically. One of my former adolescent clients, for example, would insist that he had contracted a sexually transmitted infection (even though he had not had any sexual contact with others) and pressured his parents into having him tested multiple times. Feelings of guilt can also be present, along with disrupted sleep patterns and extreme feelings of responsibility. Self-medication may also be present in adults, with alcohol and sedatives the most often abused substances (Fals-Stewart and Angarano 1994).

Conclusion

OCD is much more than just having to have things "a certain way" and is often far more impairing than how it is displayed in television shows or movies. The first step to helping someone with OCD is to understand what the disorder looks like, and this chapter should have helped you accomplish that. Despite the many problems and challenges caused by problematic obsessions and compulsions, the current outlook on OCD is much more optimistic than it was in the past (Franklin and Foa 2008). Three decades ago, OCD was considered to be a permanent, untreatable mental disorder, as there were no effective medications or therapeutic methods for this disorder at that time. Since then our understanding of both basic aspects of OCD and treatment methods has progressed to the point where OCD is now viewed as a treatable condition. A variety of empirically supported therapeutic methods and medication are available for individuals with OCD. With the proper treatment and social support, people can learn to live with and reduce their OCD symptoms.

2

POSSIBLE CAUSES OF OBSESSIVE COMPULSIVE DISORDER

Carly Johnco

Obsessive compulsive disorder (OCD) is a condition characterized by recurrent intrusive obsessions (images, thoughts, urges) and/or compulsive behaviors and rituals. Prevalence estimates of pediatric OCD suggest that this condition affects somewhere between 0.25 and 3 percent of youth. Obsessive compulsive disorder was previously classified as a type of anxiety disorder, but has most recently been classified as an independent condition under the "Obsessive-Compulsive and Related Disorders" category in the fifth version of the Diagnostic and Statistical Manual (DSM-5). It is now classed alongside conditions such as hoarding disorder, body dysmorphic disorder, trichotillomania (hair-pulling), excoriation (skin-picking) disorder, and tic disorders. This shift in categorization is the result of an increasing body of research that suggests a large amount of diagnostic and symptom overlap between these conditions. However, there is also considerable overlap and co-occurrence of OCD and anxiety disorders.

When we ask the question "What causes OCD?" we often do so with the assumption that there must be a single cause or explanation as to why a young person has developed this condition. We have all heard the rhetoric around whether it is nature vs. nurture that leads certain individuals to develop a mental illness. The implicit assumption underlying the question of causality is that if we can identify a "cause," we might be able to fix or change it, leading to a remission of symptoms, or possibly even prevention. Unfortunately, the answer to this question is not a straightforward one. The current evidence suggests that OCD is most likely to be the result of a combination of genetic, neurological, cognitive, behavioral, and environmental factors. While we are getting better at identifying certain youth who may be at an increased risk of developing OCD, at this stage, it is still very difficult to predict which children will actually develop the disorder and who will show resilience despite having increased risk in a number of domains.

This chapter will review some of the factors that have been suggested as causative or somehow implicated in the development and maintenance of OCD symptoms in youth. Rather than any single factor "causing" OCD, it is more likely that these factors increase a child's overall level of risk for developing OCD, and that certain combinations in certain children will result in the onset of a disorder. In many cases there are likely to be genetic causes and environmental causes, as well as gene-by-environmental interactions that are all involved in the onset of symptoms. Some of these risk factors are modifiable and are targeted in early intervention and treatment programs for OCD; however others (e.g., genes) cannot be altered at this stage.

Genetic factors

One of the most common assumptions for many mental health conditions, including OCD, is that they are caused by genetics, or are inherited from parents. There is some level of truth to this assumption, although this does not explain the whole picture. It is common for OCD to run in families. Family studies show OCD prevalence rates of between 7 and 15 percent in first-degree relatives of children and adolescents with OCD. Another study found that OCD was 32.5 times more common in first-degree relatives of children and adolescents with OCD than in families of youth with OCD. This familial link tends to be particularly strong amongst children who first start experiencing their OCD symptoms before the age of seven.

The question that this tends to raise is whether it is nature or nurture that explains the elevated levels of OCD in families. Do kids inherit a genetic risk for OCD, or do they "learn" their OCD symptoms from being raised around others who are affected? The answer is—potentially both. While there is substantial evidence supporting the notion that genetic factors can increase a child's vulnerability to OCD, the specific nature of *how* remains unclear. Twin studies show that it is more common for OCD concordance in monozygotic (identical) twin pairs in comparison to dizygotic (fraternal) twins, supporting the role of genetic factors in OCD. These findings suggest that the more similar your genetic makeup is to someone with OCD (as in the case of identical twins), the greater your chance of also experiencing the disorder. Heritability studies suggest that somewhere between 45 and 65 percent of the variance in childhood OCD is explained by genetic factors, with some other studies suggesting rates of up to 80 percent.

While this initially appears to be quite high, it is also important to recognize that OCD can skip generations, affect one sibling and not others, and may occur in families with no history of OCD.

While there does appear to be some increased risk for developing OCD if a family member is diagnosed, no "OCD gene" has been identified that increases a child's predisposition to the disorder, and there are a number of other factors that impact on whether a particular family member is likely to develop symptoms. The way in which genetic factors might be involved in the onset of OCD is likely to be far more complex than the way genes affect physical attributes, like height or skin color. There are a number of candidate genes that have been explored. A thorough and comprehensive review of all genes that have been explored is beyond the scope of this chapter, however most association studies have focused on genes that affect how certain chemicals (neurotransmitters) are processed in the brain. Neurons in the brain communicate by using neurotransmitters to pass messages to different parts of the brain. There are some genetic mutations that appear to affect how the brain processes these neurotransmitters, particularly genes that affect the serotonergic and dopaminergic neurotransmitter systems (e.g., mutations in the serotonin transporter gene *hSERT*, having two long alleles of the *5-HTTLPR* polymorphism, and mutations in the glutamate transporter gene *SLC1A1*). Most of the genes that have been investigated are responsible for creating the transporters that clean up and remove neurotransmitters in the synapse. Certain mutations in these genes can result in the transporter being too active, removing the neurotransmitter before it has had an opportunity to communicate with the next neuron.

Over 80 candidate genes have been investigated (e.g., *5-HTTLPR* serotonin transporter, *5HT1-D beta* serotonin receptor gene, *5HT2A* and *5HT2C* serotonin receptors, dopamine receptor type 4 (*DRD4*) gene, monoamine oxidase A (*MAO-A*), the *BDNF* locus, glutamate (*NMDA*) subunit receptor gene, overtransmission of the GABA type B receptor 1 (*GABBR1*) gene at the A-7265G polymorphism, *OLIG2*, and the myelin oligodendrocyte glycoprotein (*MOG*) gene), with most focused on serotonergic and dopaminergic pathways, however there is not enough evidence at this stage to draw any firm conclusions.

Neurobiological factors

Brain structures and functioning

Improving imaging technology and a proliferation in research has led to some interesting discoveries about certain neurobiological factors that may play a role in the development and maintenance of OCD, including both structural and functional differences in how the brain works in individuals with OCD. However, the brain is an incredibly complex organ, constantly changing and evolving, and there is still a lot that we don't know about what is going on in the brain of someone with OCD. Most of our understandings in this area come from research conducted with adults. However, there are a small number of studies that have involved children and adolescents. It can initially be an overwhelming idea that something may be wrong or different about a child's brain. It is important to remember that although the child's brain may be functioning in a way that is different, this does not mean that her symptoms are permanent. Effective psychological and pharmacological treatments are available for youth with OCD.

Brain-based research plays an important role in helping us to understand why certain symptoms occur, and is increasingly informing new research directions into the best way to directly address these symptoms. However, it is also important to interpret brain-based research with some skepticism. Most of the research that has indicated structural and functional abnormalities in OCD is conducted cross-sectionally, where individuals with OCD are compared to those without OCD at a single point in time. From a scientific perspective this can be problematic for interpreting results, because it is unclear whether youth with OCD had these types of structural and functional differences in their brain *before* developing OCD (i.e., do these neurological differences *cause* OCD?), or whether these changes in brain function occurred because of their OCD (i.e., are these changes simply reflective of the symptoms that they are *currently* experiencing?). Regardless, this research adds important pieces of information to the complex picture of understanding possible causes of OCD.

Most of the research suggests that there are three brain regions that are affected in individuals with OCD. These areas are called the cortex, striatum, and thalamus. These three regions of the brain communicate with each other via circuits referred to as cortico-striato-thalamic pathways. These pathways are part of the feedback loop between one of the deeper brain structures called the basal ganglia (responsible for coordination of movement), and regions on the surface of the brain, including the motor/premotor cortex (the area where nerve impulses for voluntary muscle movement initiate) and the orbitofrontal cortex (involved in decision-making). Research suggests that it is the *communication* between these brain regions that tends to be disrupted in individuals with OCD rather than the brain structures themselves.

Overall, these brain regions are involved in the initiation and termination of behavior. The dysfunctional communication between these structures results in youth with OCD getting "stuck" in repetitive loops of behaviors and thoughts that are difficult to stop. For example, most people wash their hands once after using the bathroom to remove any germs and then stop washing. Dysfunction in these brain circuits mean that individuals with OCD can get stuck repeating this washing process over and over, and find it difficult to "turn off" this impulse, even when they want to.

During neuropsychological testing, individuals with OCD show much greater problems than unaffected individuals in flexibly shifting away from certain patterns of thinking and in inhibiting or stopping certain patterns of behavior. Although many people will insist that a child with OCD should "snap out of it" or "just stop" what she is doing, neuroscience research has allowed us to understand that these behaviors and thoughts are not voluntary or willful actions. Certain brain functions make it difficult for individuals with OCD to stop or ignore their urges, and very difficult to disengage from these repetitive thoughts and behaviors once they begin. Many individuals with OCD will report being very frustrated and distressed by their symptoms, but feeling like they can't stop.

There is ongoing research examining a number of other brain regions (e.g., striatum, thalamus, caudate nucleus, anterior cingulate cortex, and several others) that may be involved with OCD. It is, however, not yet known exactly how differences in these brain areas might cause or affect OCD symptoms.

Neurotransmitters

In addition to these structural and functional differences, there is also evidence to suggest that individuals with OCD have abnormalities or imbalances in certain chemicals in the brain, called neurotransmitters. Neurotransmitters function like chemical signals, passing a message from one neuron to the next. The main neurotransmitter that seems to be implicated in OCD is serotonin, although there also appears to be a role for dopamine and glutamine. As discussed above, some researchers suggest that individuals with OCD show abnormalities in the way serotonin is processed in the brain. Rather than there being too much or too little of actual serotonin in the brain, the problem seems to lie in how serotonin is passed from one nerve to the next. The serotonin transporter gene hSERT is responsible for removing excess serotonin from between two synapses, and there is some recent evidence that suggests that individuals with OCD are more likely to have two mutations within this gene. This results in the transporter gene removing the serotonin from the synaptic gap before the next neuron has had a chance to receive the signal. Additional support for the potential role of neurotransmitters in OCD comes from studies that show efficacy of certain pharmacological treatments for the treatment of OCD, namely selective serotonin reuptake inhibitors (SSRIs). These medications target this serotonin transporter gene to allow the serotonin to stay in the synapse a little longer to allow the chemical message to be passed along.

The role of the neurotransmitter glutamate is less well understood, although some studies have discovered that abnormal levels have been found amongst patients with OCD. For example, increased levels of glutamate have been found in the cerebrospinal fluid of some people with OCD, and other studies have found decreased levels in certain brain regions.

The role of dopamine in OCD is also complex. There appears to be a link between the decreased levels of serotonin in the cortico-striato-thalamic pathway and increased levels of dopamine in the prefrontal cortex. Dopamine is the neurotransmitter associated with reward pathways and reward-motivated behavior. In OCD, compulsions become associated with a reduction in anxiety over time, and can be triggered by some level of pleasure-seeking. Rodent research has shown that stimulating the dopamine receptors can result in OCD-like behaviors in rats. Indirect support for the role of dopamine in OCD has also come from the efficacy of some pharmacological agents that control dopamine activity. However, there are a large number of studies that have not found any differences in the amount of dopamine (its metabolites) in youth with OCD compared to unaffected children. Despite inconsistencies in the literature, there is, in general, evidence to suggest some associations with dopamine neurotransmission and OCD symptoms.

Autoimmunity

Pediatric Acute-onset Neuropsychiatric Syndrome (PANS) is a syndrome where youth experience a particularly abrupt (often overnight) onset of OCD and/or tic symptoms, often accompanied by other neuropsychiatric symptoms such as restricted eating, anxiety, significant declines in handwriting and math abilities, increased urinary frequency, and sensory hypersensitivity. Youth with PANS experience an acute onset of OCD or tic symptoms before puberty, and tend to experience relapsing-remitting course of symptoms. The exact cause of PANS is unknown, however is thought to be the result of infection, metabolic problems, or a misdirected inflammatory reaction that affects the brain. Over a decade of research focused on Streptococcal infection as the underlying cause of these rapid-onset symptoms, and these children were diagnosed with Pediatric Autoimmune Neuropsychiatric Disorders Associated with Streptococcal Infections (PANDAS). Although PANDAS was identified long before PANS, it is now considered a subtype of PANS. Group A streptococcal infections can cause inflammation in the basal ganglia, a region of the brain heavily implicated in OCD symptoms (see above).

Controversy as to the etiology of these rapid-onset cases of OCD prompted the introduction of the PANS diagnosis in 2012 to accommodate youth who had similar phenotypic symptoms, but had negative test results for the Streptococcal infection. Although a Group A Streptococcal infection is not required for PANS diagnosis, most cases show some temporal association with this infection and symptom onset or exacerbation. There is still a need for more research to understand why some youth experience PANS; however a number of other potential triggers have been identified, including Lyme's disease, H1N1 virus, and certain microorganisms in the gut following prophylactic antibiotic treatment. Hallmark features of youth with PANS include neurological abnormalities, particularly choreiform movements (a repetitive, jerky, and involuntary movement), and a notable regression in handwriting and math abilities.

Cognitive causes of OCD

In addition to the above biological factors, there are a number of psychological and environmental factors that appear to play a role in the development of OCD. Youth with OCD tend to make a number of characteristic errors in the way they think about and interpret information that can lead to obsessive thinking styles and subsequent compulsive behaviors. Intrusive thoughts are a common experience that most people disregard relatively quickly as unimportant. However, youth with OCD typically inflate the importance of these thoughts. For youth with OCD, the mere presence of these thoughts can be interpreted as dangerous, harmful, or threatening. As such, individuals often experience a high level of anxiety (and in many cases shame, embarrassment, or disgust depending on the content of the intrusive thought), and engage in a range of behaviors in an attempt to neutralize the perceived threat. Individuals often describe their compulsions as a way of "undoing" the danger that arises from their intrusive thoughts. For example, a child with OCD may have a thought or image about her parent being in a car accident, and that as a result of having this thought, she has increased the risk that her parent will actually be in an accident. In order to "un-do" the danger that her thought has created for the parent, the child may count to a special number or perform a particular touching ritual. She will often describe that this behavior (magically) protects her parent from harm, or takes away the danger that she created.

There are six ways that individuals with OCD commonly misinterpret their thoughts. These patterns ultimately contribute to and maintain their OCD symptoms:

- *Inflated responsibility*—when individuals believe that they are personally responsible for preventing negative outcomes from occurring.

- *Over-importance of thoughts*—when individuals believe that having certain thoughts increases the probability of a negative event occurring. In the case of intrusive thoughts about behaviors or actions, this can also refer to the individual believing that having the thought is morally equivalent to actually engaging in the behavior. This is often referred to as "magical thinking" given the inherent implausibility or superstition surrounding this logic.

- *Excessive concern about controlling one's thoughts*—individuals with OCD often believe that it is important and possible to "control" their thoughts. This drive to suppress or control unwanted thoughts usually leads to an increase in the frequency of the thoughts. There are decades of research suggesting that suppression of thoughts generally leads to a rebound effect, where the frequency of the thoughts actually increases.

- *Overestimation of threat*—individuals with OCD often overestimate the likelihood of danger, as well as having an inflated belief about how catastrophic an event will be if it occurs (i.e., it is very likely that [negative outcome] will happen, and if it does it will be [catastrophic]).

- *Intolerance of uncertainty*—a belief that the individual needs to know, without any doubt, that negative events will not occur.

- *Perfectionism*—a belief that everything needs to perfect, and an excessive concern about making mistakes.

Behavioral causes of OCD

Behavioral models and theories of OCD suggest that individuals learn to associate certain objects with fear. Avoidance of things that trigger fear or anxiety is a natural response, designed to help us steer clear of danger. However, in the case of OCD, the avoidance becomes excessive given the objective level of danger. Although avoidance reduces anxiety in the short term, it ultimately increases anxiety in the longer term because the individual never gets to learn that nothing bad happens, and that she can tolerate the situation/her distress. Individuals with OCD often develop certain rituals that function to help them avoid or neutralize situations that trigger their anxiety. Over time, a cycle of avoidance and rituals develops, strengthening the anxiety. For example, a child may at some stage make a connection between toilets and germs (a link often directly articulated to youth). The child may begin to avoid touching toilets for fear of being exposed to the germs. Over time this may generalize to avoidance of touching other "dirty" objects (e.g., doorknobs, toys, food, other people). This avoidance strengthens her fear of germs, and often leads to an increased preoccupation with having been exposed to contaminants. Commonly, these concerns about having been exposed to contaminants leads to an increase in rituals surrounding washing and decontamination. Engaging in avoidance and rituals may decrease anxiety in the short term, but ultimately increases her anxiety and fear during subsequent encounters with the same (or similar) situations.

Environmental causes of OCD

As discussed above, there are a number of biological and genetic factors that may increase a child's risk of developing OCD. However, the presence of these factors alone is often not sufficient to result in OCD. Some environmental factors appear to also increase the risk of OCD, with the interaction between biological, psychological, and environmental triggers most likely to explain the onset of OCD. Twin studies suggest that environmental factors account for between 20 and 41 percent of the variance in obsessive compulsive behaviors, although others suggest that this rate may be much higher (between 53 and 73 percent). Although some studies have failed to find this association, there are a number of studies that have found higher levels of exposure to traumatic and stressful life events amongst individuals with OCD (e.g., abuse, bereavement, bullying, parental conflict or divorce, and illness), especially in the few years before their symptoms started. Similarly, exposure to stressful events can exacerbate symptoms in children who are already affected by OCD.

Although higher rates of exposure to these events have been documented in youth with OCD, stressful life events are unlikely to cause OCD on their own. Stress is more likely to make a child more vulnerable to OCD when she already has a number of other risk factors. To be clichéd, stress may be the "straw that breaks the camel's back" for some kids. The exception to this may be in the case of traumatic brain injuries, where higher rates of obsessive thoughts and behaviors are often noted as a result of structural brain damage.

One of the most influential environmental factors for pediatric OCD is the role of families. Families can play an important role in how children learn about fear and safety. In the case of children being raised in an environment with an affected family member they may be at an increased genetic risk. However, these children are also exposed to certain OCD behaviors that they accidentally learn from via parent modeling. For example, a parent with contamination fears may repeatedly wash her own hands. However, she is also likely to repetitively clean the child's hands and/or scold her for touching "dirty" objects. Children learn by watching others, and may learn to mimic these washing (or other) rituals, as well as internalizing certain obsessional beliefs. For example, a child who sees a parent check the locks on the house over and over again may internalize this fear, and also develop compulsive checking behaviors. In this way, family members can inadvertently reinforce certain OCD symptoms in a child.

Another way that family can unintentionally contribute to OCD symptoms is that they begin to play a role in the child's avoidance/ritual cycle, something referred to as family accommodation. In the case of OCD, families often end up involved in the child's OCD symptoms and rituals in some way. This can include participating in certain compulsions and rituals, facilitating avoidance of certain anxiety-provoking objects/situations, providing reassurance, or altering the child's or family routine because of the child's OCD symptoms. In almost all cases, families do this in an attempt to reduce the child's distress (and perhaps their own as well). For example, in response to a child's requests, or in anticipation of the child becoming worried about germs, a parent may wash her hands with increased frequency before touching the child's belongings, launder the child's towel and clothes daily, and purchase antibacterial wash or excessive quantities of soap. Other examples of accommodation that are common in parents of youth with OCD can include counting to special numbers with a child, doing things in a particular order dictated by the child's OCD, and altering the family routine (e.g., leaving early/late to accommodate a ritual) to appease the child. Unfortunately, although these accommodations may help to temporarily reduce the child's discomfort, it ultimately feeds back into the avoidance cycle of anxiety and increases her distress in the long term. When individuals with OCD engage in avoidance and/or rituals, they do not have the opportunity to learn that they can tolerate the situation.

3

THE DEVELOPMENT AND COURSE OF CHILDHOOD OBSESSIVE COMPULSIVE DISORDER

Dean McKay

According to the World Health Organization (WHO), obsessive compulsive disorder (OCD) is among the top ten disabling illnesses (Markarian *et al.* 2010). The disorder is characterized by frequent intrusive and unwanted thoughts or images that typically cause anxiety. Compulsions often develop as a means to interrupt or prevent the intrusive thoughts and images. In general individuals will also avoid situations that may provoke obsessions. In most cases, individuals recognize the senselessness of symptoms (APA 2013).

Family members and friends may be recruited to assist in alleviating the obsessions. This can be accomplished in several ways. One way is through reassurance that the obsessions are not valid or are gross exaggerations of perceived danger associated with the thought. Another is by participation in the compulsions, such as doing specific activities repeatedly. Finally, individuals with OCD may request assistance in avoidance of situations that would give rise to the obsessions.

Children with OCD may present with a range of symptoms that are highly variable. One major measure of symptoms in childhood OCD, the Children's Yale-Brown Obsessive–Compulsive Scale, includes the following broad categories of symptoms on the checklist: obsessions associated with contamination, aggression, sexual behavior, magical ideation/superstitions, somatic concerns, religion, and hoarding, as well as items concerning compulsions for washing, checking, repeating, ordering/arranging, and rituals involving other people. It is common for children to have symptoms of OCD in multiple categories (i.e., obsessions regarding contamination in addition to magical ideation/superstitions) (McKay *et al.* 2006).

Contemporary treatment for childhood OCD emphasizes exposure and response prevention (ERP) along with family and/or caregiver involvement in order to (a) ensure that interventions are carried out between sessions following development and practice within session, and (b) to decrease the degree that family members accommodate for the child's symptoms (Franklin *et al.* 2015). Accommodation has been found to be an important specific contributor to childhood symptoms, whereby caregivers or family members effectively participate in the child's symptoms, aid in avoidance, or provide a wide range of reassurance, all of which contributes to the perpetuation of symptoms (Lebowitz, Scharfstein, and Jones 2014).

Cognitive behavioral therapy (CBT) employing ERP focuses on gradually and progressively exposing the affected child to objects or situations that might give rise to obsessions, with corresponding blockage of rituals. The first step, following the intake assessment, is the development of a hierarchy of feared objects and/or situations. This hierarchy serves as the basis for how treatment progresses, since it provides a guideline for how exposure may be conducted, beginning with easier items and moving up to more challenging ones. This method requires that, in addition to focusing on the primary feared areas, the therapist also emphasizes the positives associated with success and reinforces the child for moving through the items. The notion of rewarding the child for progressing through exposure exercises allows for two specific processes to unfold. First, and in keeping with the aim of exposure, the child gains mastery over feared situations through habituation and naturally occurring corrective information regarding the dangerousness of the object or situation (Foa and Kozak 1986). More recent conceptualizations of the mechanisms of action underlying exposure emphasize a wide range of additional learning including changing expectations and reinforcement for practicing exposure (Craske *et al.* 2014). This more recent conceptualization, referred to as the inhibitory learning model, stresses a range of other clinical approaches that may be employed to facilitate fear reduction associated with a wide range of anxiety problems. In the case of children these additional methods are particularly salient given the inherent challenge in engaging a fearful child in activities that, by ordinary description, may seem to have the potential to increase fear. Despite this, when done properly, many children are capable of engaging in ERP, and treatment outcome is generally favorable (Franklin *et al.* 2015).

In addition to CBT, pharmacotherapy is commonly employed to treat children with OCD. The most widely accepted and efficacious treatment for childhood OCD is selective serotonin reuptake inhibitor (SSRI) medication

(Ivarsson *et al.* 2015). This approach to treatment has a hypothesized mechanism of action on specific neural components of repetitive actions and ideas associated with OCD that in turn activate a putative fear circuit (Abramowitz, Taylor, and McKay 2009). It has been shown that SSRI pharmacotherapy alleviates symptoms, but to a lesser degree than CBT (Ivarsson *et al.* 2015). Further, SSRI medications have well known risks, namely increased suicidal ideation in adolescence (McCain 2009). As a result, it is often recommended that treatment with medication is accompanied by CBT (Ivarsson *et al.* 2015).

Age of onset and epidemiology

OCD was once considered a rare condition, but also the subject of intense interest among clinicians. While Janet (1903) discussed obsessive compulsive symptoms and described psychopathological features that defined the disorder, Freud provided one of the first clinical accounts in his famous case of the Rat Man, where a young man experienced disabling intrusive images that rats would consume his father and girlfriend. In the modern era of psychiatry, our understanding of the rate of OCD and ability to inquire sensitively regarding the symptoms has shown that OCD is a highly prevalent condition. Most estimates of the prevalence of OCD in the general population is 2 to 3 percent, with most cases developing before the age of 25 (Samuels and Nestadt 1997), although some estimates have been as high as 14.7 percent using a school sample (Alvarenga *et al.* 2015). It has been reported that, if untreated, the course of the disorder is stable, meaning that spontaneous remission is rare. While research on remission rates have been sparse, estimates of complete symptom alleviation following treatment are between 10 and 15 percent (Zohar 1999). Epidemiology research also suggests that OCD is highly comorbid with other psychiatric conditions, with fewer than a quarter of cases being solely diagnosed with the condition (Snider and Swedo 2000). Among the most common comorbid conditions are tic disorders, major depression, and developmental disorders. Given the high rate of comorbid tic disorders, several studies have evaluated the prevalence in conjunction with this additional diagnostic category. Research has suggested that presence of tics and/or OCD in families substantially increases the risk of the disorder in offspring (Browne *et al.* 2015). Finally, research has suggested that age of onset for OCD is earlier in boys than girls (Zohar 1999), although overall slightly more females than males come down with the disorder (Craske 2003).

Models of etiology

Treatment of any condition proceeds most efficiently when there are sound and testable conceptualizations of etiology and maintenance. The dominant areas of research related to etiology and maintenance of OCD fall generally into heritability (or genetic), biological, learning, and cognitive. The investigations into these models are derived from basic laboratory research or treatment trials.

Heritability

It has long been suggested that OCD runs in families, but as with all research involving heredity, it is a challenge to separate environmental influences from biological ones. Overall, research suggests that OCD runs in families

(Browne *et al.* 2014). For example, one study found a three-fold increase in risk for OCD if a family member has OCD (Black *et al.* 2013). In another investigation that was multigenerational in nature, a 2.6 times greater risk was found for OCD in families with at least one affected member, even if it was an individual two generations previous (Mataix-Cols *et al.* 2013). As a result, it appears that OCD risk is increased when a family member has the condition. However, this line of research has not adequately addressed whether the risk is due to observing someone exhibit the behaviors or the disorder, or a result of a biological risk factor.

Turning to the biomedical risk research, genetic research has not yet turned up any strong associations. One major approach to identifying genes (or combinations of genes) related to a condition is a methodology referred to as a genome wide association study (GWAS). In this approach to genetic research, a set of individuals with a known condition has their entire genome mapped, and these genomes are then compared to a group without the condition under study. In a major GWAS on OCD, Stewart *et al.* (2013) did not identify any genes or combinations of genes associated with the disorder. Prior to the development of the GWAS methodology, there were a large number of laboratory based gene-specific investigations of OCD. These studies evaluated hypothesized genes for their association with OCD (such as genes related to serotonin, dopamine, or catecholemines). In a meta-analysis of the data from these studies, Taylor (2013) found that OCD likely involves several genes that individually do not contribute much to the onset of OCD, but only when present collectively does the risk of the disorder increase significantly. According to the analysis by

Taylor, genes related to serotonin, dopamine, and glutamate collectively increase the odds of an individual developing OCD, but even in this case the increased risk was only 1.4 times greater than if this collection of genes were not present. This is a low genetic risk overall. In fact, genetics researchers have suggested that a minimum increased risk of 2.5 times greater than without the gene be the threshold for declaring that a psychiatric condition is heritable (Kendler 2005). As a result, it is best to conclude, at the present time, that genetic research has not yet identified a gene or set of genes that is associated with OCD.

Biological models of etiology

OCD has long been considered a biologically based illness, with the neurotransmitter serotonin implicated in the condition (Gross *et al.* 1998). The fundamental notion underlying the serotonin hypothesis has been that the neurotransmitter does not remain in the synaptic cleft for sufficient durations, or that there are insufficient levels of serotonin overall. Given that there are brain areas where serotonin is particularly prominent, ones associated with judgment, decision-making, and emotional arousal, this hypothesis has been a dominant component of medical treatment for OCD. Further, as serotonin is also implicated in depression (Albert, Benkelfat, and Descarries 2012), this hypothesis has served as a useful bridge between these two conditions. The serotonin hypothesis has been useful as a means for the development and administration of a wide range of SSRI medications, which are among the most widely prescribed for OCD, and have accumulated the greatest empirical support for their efficacy, including in children (Ivarsson *et al.* 2015).

While serotonin has been an important neurotransmitter in understanding the biological basis of OCD, treatment outcomes with SSRI medications have failed to provide sufficient relief to sufferers. This has led to researchers investigating other neurotransmitters that could reasonably be implicated in OCD. At this time, the research on these other neurotransmitters is still in development, with few conclusions that can be reasonably drawn.

NEURAL CIRCUITRY

Currently there is an emphasis on a network of brain areas that, collectively, lead to obsessive compulsive symptoms. These brain networks, or circuits (described in Insel *et al.* 2010) have been examined using brain imaging methods (such as functional magnetic resonance imaging). In the case of OCD, the circuit that has been described centers on areas related to judgment and decision-making (orbitofrontal cortex), response inhibition (dorsolateral prefrontal cortex), emotional response (substantia nigra and globus pallidus), and repetitive actions (basal ganglia system) (Abramowitz *et al.* 2009). On the one hand, there is emerging evidence in basic laboratory research of a brain circuit system in OCD (Piras *et al.* 2015). That is, the circuits appear active in individuals with the diagnosis. However, if these brain circuits are in fact associated with the disorder, then changes in the circuitry should be evident in treatment. On this latter note, the research is mixed, with some studies showing a strong association with treatment and others demonstrating no role for these brain areas in association with therapy (McKay and Tolin 2016). In one review, it appeared that changes in brain circuitry with treatment was highly specific, with therapy benefiting dorsal brain areas (i.e., basal ganglia) during symptom provocation, and also benefiting ventral circuits (i.e., prefrontal cortex areas) during cognitive processing of information (Thorsen, van den Heuvel, and Hansen 2015).

NEUROPSYCHOLOGY

Neuropsychological research involves primarily indirect assessments, using memory, decision-making, and other tests that are correlated with a broad range of brain functions. To this end, OCD has been a source of considerable investigation employing neuropsychological tests, in an effort to identify potential areas of function, and by extension brain areas, that may be involved in the disorder.

Broadly speaking, it appears that several conclusions may be drawn regarding OCD. First, OCD is associated with problems in organizational memory, which draws on orbitofrontal cortex functioning in conjunction with temporal lobe processing (Greisberg and McKay 2003). More recent research has suggested that neuropsychological research in OCD demonstrates problems in three broad areas of functioning: executive functioning efficiency, task complexity, and memory load (Harkin and Kessler 2011). In a recent quantitative summary of the available neuropsychology literature, broad executive functioning deficits were observed in OCD (Snyder *et al.* 2015). In the case of children, the research on neuropsychological function lags behind that for adults. Unlike in the adult literature, a systematic review of neuropsychological test results does not suggest deficits in any areas of functioning (Abramovitch *et al.* 2015). Despite this, one recent investigation found that there were differences in neuropsychology test performance in children with OCD based on primary symptoms, with those exhibiting hoarding or symmetry/ordering symptoms showing the highest level of deficits on measures of executive functioning or memory (McGuire *et al.* 2014).

While several reviews have pointed to deficit areas in adult OCD, and no significant effects in children, it has also been noted that many neuropsychology tests lack predictive utility (or ecological validity), and that investigators need to identify assessment areas that capture the kinds of executive and memory deficits evident in OCD that are germane to the everyday lives of sufferers (Abramovitch and Cooperman 2015).

Cognitive behavioral models of etiology

The biological perspective has informed a great deal of conceptualization and treatment of OCD. Psychosocial approaches have largely centered on behavioral theory (notably learning theory) and cognitive theory.

LEARNING

Learning theory has suggested that OCD can develop in susceptible individuals. This perspective on the disorder has been fundamental in the development of efficacious treatment, namely exposure and response prevention (ERP) (McKay *et al.* 2015). This approach to treatment assumes that situations that provoke obsessions are learned through classical conditioning, and can therefore be alleviated (extinguished) by repeated exposure without the feared consequences.

The original conceptualization of classical condition emphasized neural associations formed as part of the learning experience. The neural basis of learning has been the foundation for recent research on "cognitive enhancers," medications that, when used in conjunction with extinction-based treatments such as ERP, facilitate outcome. Research using one of these cognitive enhancers, d-cycloserine, suggests that extinction may be hastened in the treatment of childhood OCD when ERP is applied (Byrne *et al.* 2015), which would lead to better treatment outcomes. On the other hand, if OCD symptoms are learned responses, it should also be the case that individuals with the disorder would show faster rates of fear learning compared to individuals who do not have the disorder. Recent research has supported this hypothesis in youth (McGuire *et al.* 2016), although there was no difference in the rate of extinction compared to control participants.

Basic learning theory has been highly influential in fostering treatments that alleviate symptoms of OCD. Nonetheless, there remain important ways in which these treatments fall short of addressing maintaining features of the condition. To illustrate, many individuals with OCD report non fear-based responses to exposure, such as disgust (Olatunji and McKay 2007). It has been shown that these other emotional responses do not necessarily respond as quickly to exposure, if at all (McKay 2006). These other reactions have been accounted for by a modification of learning theory called evaluative conditioning (EC). The essential basis for EC is that in conjunction with original classical conditioning, the respondent also labels the experience in an emotionally toned manner (i.e., "that's yucky"). Once such a label is applied, it becomes more difficult to apply extinction-based methods (such as ERP; Mason and Richardson 2012). This perspective has been considered a central method of learning for contamination fear in OCD in particular (Ludvik, Boschen, and Neuman 2015).

SITUATIONAL AND COGNITIVE APPRAISAL

The EC model opens the door for evaluations of a wide range of circumstances by an individual with OCD other than those in classical conditioning situations. Broadly speaking, the cognitive model has gained prominence, originating with the work of Salkovskis (1985). Specifically, this framework posits that individuals with OCD appraise situations along specific dimensions such as degree of responsibility for thoughts that might be associated with harm (Salkovskis 1985). Since then, the cognitive model has been expanded to include a wide range of common situational appraisals, including perfectionism, over importance of thoughts, overestimation of threat, and intolerance of uncertainty. These thought domains have not been well investigated in children despite it being hypothesized as central to the disorder. There have been some retrospective reports, which have been suggestive of a relationship (i.e., Yarbro *et al.* 2013), but these suffer from problems of participant emotional state during completion of the measures and accuracy of memory for events.

The cognitive model is compelling, however, because many individuals with OCD report patterns of thinking that conform to the beliefs described here. While this is an important consideration, research has not shown these beliefs to show several key features that would make the model a strong framework for understanding the etiology and maintenance of the condition. That is, the available research has not shown that the cognitive model has *generality* (or applicability to the full range of symptoms for the condition), *specificity* (or associated with OCD over and above other conditions), and *congruence* (or associated to specific symptoms in a meaningful way) (Tolin, Worhunsky, and Maltby 2006). Based on the available evidence, it would appear that obsessive compulsive beliefs are chiefly useful in conceptualization of patterns of thinking that foster anxious responses generally, but not OCD in particular. This conclusion is drawn from research showing that the beliefs associated with OCD are also present in other anxiety disorders (Taylor *et al.* 2006) and that the core hypothesized belief domains for OCD are primarily associated with less severe symptoms (Kim *et al.* 2016).

Depression in OCD

Many individuals who suffer from OCD also struggle with depressed mood. The challenge for investigators and clinicians is discerning the degree that the depression is a consequence of the OCD (secondary) or emerged as a syndrome in its own right separate from OCD (comorbid). This is important as treatment decisions may be made to address OCD symptoms if it is assessed that the depression is a consequence of the disorder, but depression may be directly targeted if it is deemed comorbid. Research has consistently suggested that comorbid depression is a poor prognostic indicator for OCD treatment (Keeley *et al.* 2008). Recent research with children has suggested that comorbidity is not the problem per se in determining illness risk for OCD. Instead, the propensity for experiencing depressed mood, whether a result of OCD or not, was predictive of poorer treatment outcome, and of requiring a lengthier course of treatment (Nissen, Nikolajsen, and Thomsen 2014).

Clinical course of OCD

The earliest clinical descriptions of OCD came from Janet (1903), who articulated basic features of the problem and suggested that it was comprised of problems in affective responding, perceptual challenges such as persistent feelings of incompleteness, depersonalization, derealization, and a broad deficit in psychological mindedness. All of these problems were considered central psychological challenges that, if left unaddressed, would also leave the sufferer impaired with symptoms. Around the time of Janet, Freud was likewise offering a conceptual account of obsessionality. According to Freud, obsessional experiences were associated with restricting emotional reactions, concealing the concerns from view, and as a result it was thought there were far more sufferers from obsessional experiences than appeared for treatment (Freud 1895).

Long-term studies evaluating individuals with OCD suggest a chronic course of illness, with males showing greater morbidity and poorer outcomes in treatment (Sharma, Thennarasu, and Reddy 2014). This study further showed that an earlier age of onset, duration of illness, and severity were predictive of poorer long-term outcome and chronicity of course. While epidemiology research suggests that more women are diagnosed with OCD, men fare poorer in long-term treatment and have more frequent return of symptoms (Torresan et al. 2013). Finally, it was found that over time individuals with OCD tend to accumulate additional psychiatric diagnoses, contributing further to the long-term morbidity of the condition (Yaryura-Tobias et al. 2000).

Specific symptoms have been shown to substantially influence the course of the illness. For example, concerns with symmetry tend to be associated with an earlier age of onset, and harming related thoughts tend to wax and wane across the lifespan (Kichuk *et al.* 2013). Further, individuals with comorbid obsessive compulsive personality disorder have been found to be at greater risk of relapse following successful treatment whereas those with harming obsessions alone were most likely to experience full relief from symptoms (Eisen *et al.* 2013). Finally, it has been shown that specific symptoms are more responsive to treatment than others. Notably, symmetry/ordering obsessions and contamination obsessions are most responsive to treatment, whereas checking responds less well to intervention, and hoarding (which is no longer formerly within OCD but is instead an obsessive compulsive related disorder) responds poorest (Abramowitz *et al.* 2003).

Overall, the research on clinical course of OCD suggests a complex etiology, with outcome dependent on several critical patient factors. First, males appear to require specific attention in treatment to ensure long-term efficacious outcome. Second, left untreated, OCD tends to not only worsen, but the prospect for benefit from treatment tends to worsen with time. Third, the presence of personality disorders, particularly obsessive compulsive personality, tends to aggravate outcome and increases the risk of relapse.

Conclusion

There are a wide range of factors that contribute to the onset and maintenance of OCD. Further, the disorder is highly complex and heterogeneous, meaning that there is a wide range of putative models that account for the disorder, with no single framework established with dominant empirical support. At the present time, there is a great deal of investigative work being done to evaluating biological mechanisms of the disorder, while at the same time there is solid evidence supporting the cognitive-behavioral model. The cognitive–behavioral model has resulted in promising treatment, but the availability of this approach is still limited due to a variety of training and clinician receptivity to ERP (McKay *et al.* 2015). With the advent of new standards for empirically supported treatments (Tolin *et al.* 2015) and emerging clinical practice guidelines (Hollon *et al.* 2014), it is anticipated that these highly effective treatments will become more widely available to clients who have the misfortune of being geographically remote from a competent provider. With the increased access to care, it is also anticipated that research will deepen our understanding of the putative developmental factors that contribute to this disorder.

Just over 50 years ago, it was thought that not only was OCD completely refractory to treatment, but that efforts to intervene in the condition would only lead to symptom exacerbation (Kringlen 1965). The field has come a considerable way from that time, where now OCD sufferers are far more likely to not only find relief, but have effective treatment options including SSRI medication, ERP, or cognitive therapy. Nonetheless, the clinical course of the disorder reveals that while many sufferers find relief, there is a high likelihood of symptom remission, requiring that once the diagnosis is conferred sufferers and their families remain vigilant for indicators of a return of illness. Early detection and treatment are clearly vital, and as a result, interventions aimed at children with the nascent signs of the disorder are key to alleviating the symptoms and increasing the odds that the condition will remain at bay.

4

RECOGNIZING OBSESSIVE COMPULSIVE DISORDER

Marni L. Jacob

Obsessive compulsive disorder (OCD) is a fairly common neuropsychiatric disorder affecting children and adolescents. Obsessions are recurrent intrusive thoughts, images, or impulses that cause significant distress. Compulsions are ritualistic behaviors that are often performed in efforts to reduce distress and/or prevent something bad from happening. The presence of OCD is often associated with significant distress and interference with child and family functioning. Youth with OCD may also present with different clinical profiles depending on their age at the time of evaluation. Accordingly, it is important for children, parents, and professionals to be knowledgeable about how to identify OCD symptoms, as proper identification of symptoms will facilitate effective intervention. However, there are many challenges to identification of OCD symptoms. Parents may find themselves wondering whether particular behaviors they observe are conceptualized as OCD symptoms, or whether they are simply normal, developmentally appropriate behaviors. For example, children may exhibit a preference for lining up Lego bricks or organizing dolls in a particular manner, and such behavior would be unlikely to be classified as OCD unless the behaviors were distressing and interfering with the child's functioning. Further, given the significant symptom overlap between OCD and other psychological disorders (e.g., anxiety, Tourette Syndrome), it may also be hard to determine how symptoms are best classified. This chapter provides guidance to help children, parents, and professionals recognize OCD. It also includes particular factors to keep in mind in the assessment of OCD.

Common themes in pediatric OCD

When conducting a thorough assessment of OCD symptoms, it is particularly helpful to have a good understanding of common themes often present in OCD. Knowledge of such themes provides a starting point during the assessment process. A discussion of common themes can also be a way to normalize OCD symptoms so the youth is more apt to disclose symptoms. The following section describes several of the themes often present in pediatric OCD.

Aggressive obsessions

Symptoms may include a fear that the individual might harm herself, fear that she might harm others, violent or horrific images, fear of doing something embarrassing, fear that she will act on unwanted impulses (e.g., stabbing someone, pushing someone off a ledge), fear that she will steal things, fear of accidentally harming others (e.g., hit/run), or a fear that she'll be responsible for something bad happening (e.g., fire/burglary). Youth may engage in significant avoidance of things that trigger these thoughts to reduce the likelihood of acting impulsively (e.g., avoiding use of sharp objects).

Checking behaviors

Such symptoms may include checking locks, stove, appliances, checking that the child did not or will not harm herself or others, checking that nothing terrible did or will happen, checking that she didn't make a mistake (e.g., excessive checking of schoolwork), and mental analyzing or checking behaviors (e.g., reviewing conversations in her head).

Contamination concerns

Youth may experience concern or disgust with bodily waste or secretions (e.g., urine, feces, saliva, blood), excessive concern with dirt or germs, excessive concern with environmental contaminants (e.g., asbestos, radiation), excessive concern with household items (e.g., cleansers, chemicals), excessive concern with animals (e.g., insects), concerns that they will become sick because of germs/contaminants, concerns that they will spread contaminants and get others sick, concerns with how it will feel to be contaminated (e.g., feeling dirty, experiencing disgust), and being bothered by sticky substances or residues. Common compulsions include excessive or ritualized hand washing, showering, bathing, teeth brushing, grooming, or toilet routine, excessive cleaning of household items or other objects, and excessive measures to prevent or remove contact with contaminants (e.g., using a towel to open a bathroom door). For some, contamination-related OCD symptoms may also have a basis in an over-reactive response to disgust, suggesting that those with OCD may have a hypersensitivity to the emotion of disgust (e.g., thinking one's hands feel disgusting unless they are washed).

Counting symptoms

Youth may engage in a variety of counting rituals, such as counting while engaging in compulsive behaviors (e.g., counting to a certain number while washing or checking), counting various items (e.g., floor or ceiling tiles), and counting actions (e.g., steps taken).

"Just right" obsessions and need for symmetry or exactness

Youth may experience thoughts that things have to be in the right place or else something bad could happen, or feelings that things have to be a certain way or "just right" or else the child experiences distress. Youth may engage in a behavior with one hand and will feel an uncomfortable tactile sensation until they do the same behavior with the other hand to make things "even." They may report that things feel "wrong" unless they are done a particular way. These symptoms may also involve compulsions in which a child feels the urge to touch, tap, or rub things in a particular way.

Ordering/organizing/arranging symptoms

Such symptoms may include thoughts that things (e.g., clothes, books) have to be organized perfectly, or else it may interfere with functioning, as well as urges to organize alphabetically, by color, or by size. Youth may feel that their backpack or desk needs to be arranged a certain way in order for them to feel better.

Religious obsessions/scrupulosity

These symptoms may include excessive concern with sacrilege and blasphemy, fear of offending God, fear of going to hell, excessive concern with right and wrong, and a heightened sense of morality. Obsessions may be associated with excessive prayer, reassurance-seeking behavior, and confessing of obsessive thoughts.

Repeating rituals

Common repeating rituals include re-reading, erasing, and re-writing, and a need to repeat routine activities (e.g., going in and out of the door).

Sexual obsessions

Symptoms may include unwanted forbidden or perverse sexual thoughts, images, or impulses; intrusive sexual thoughts involving children or incest; intrusive sexual thoughts with content involving homosexuality; and intrusive thoughts of aggressive sexual behavior towards others (e.g., molestation, sexual violence). Youth with these thoughts may engage in efforts to try to suppress these thoughts, or avoid situations or places (e.g., playground, "R" rated movies) that trigger these thoughts, given that such thoughts are unpleasant and unwanted. These symptoms may be particularly challenging to identify given that children may be embarrassed and reluctant to even admit that they are experiencing such thoughts. For instance, the youth may fear repercussions such as a getting into trouble. Despite the often taboo nature of these thoughts, their unpleasant and unwanted nature, combined with the fact that such thoughts are often associated with compulsions (e.g., avoidance, confessing) highlights that the child is likely not at risk for engaging in such behaviors. It is also important to note that these thoughts are irrational in nature, and do not necessarily indicate that the youth was exposed to any previous trauma.

Somatic obsessions

Youth may experience excessive concern with illness or disease, or excessive concern with a body part or an aspect of appearance. Children may repetitively seek reassurance from parents or doctors, and they may engage in checking tied to somatic obsessions.

Magical thinking/superstitious fears

Magical thinking and superstitious fears are particularly common among children with OCD. This may include the belief in lucky or unlucky numbers, or avoidance of colors with special significance. Children may feel that they have to avoid walking on cracks in order to prevent something bad from happening. In magical thinking in OCD, a child may perceive two events that are unrelated as being related in some manner. For example, a child may have the thought that unless she performs a ritual (e.g., saying a phrase), something bad could happen to someone she cares about (e.g., involvement in a car accident).

Miscellaneous symptoms

A variety of other symptoms may also manifest in youth with OCD. Examples of such symptoms include a need to know or remember, fear of saying certain things, fear of not saying just the right thing, or a fear of losing things. Such symptoms may then be associated with rituals such as reassurance-seeking behavior. Youth may also experience intrusive nonsense sounds, words, or music, or be excessively bothered by certain sounds or noises. Other compulsions may include excessive list making, blinking or staring rituals, and ritualized eating behaviors.

Factors to consider in assessment

An assessment of pediatric OCD should include a comprehensive evaluation of current and past OCD symptoms, symptom severity, avoidance, and associated functional impairment. The particular fears and beliefs underlying the obsessions should be clearly detailed, along with the compulsive behaviors that are performed in an effort to reduce anxiety. In young children, compulsions without obsessions can be more common. Avoidance occurs when the child with OCD seeks to evade the situations that she feels trigger her OCD. Avoidance is her way of trying to prevent the distress that would be associated with coming into contact with the trigger, or prevent the extensive rituals that she would feel compelled to perform. A child may say she is "not hungry" when presented with a food that she perceives might be contaminated or might refuse to get dressed to avoid going to a location she perceives to be risky. The presence (or worsening) of OCD symptoms may also become more apparent because of physical markers (e.g., dry, chafed skin in those with excessive hand washing), increased use of soap/cleaning products, "vanishing" toilet paper (from excessive wiping), changing clothes frequently, or increasing water bills.

When conducting the initial assessment, it may be helpful to spend some time interviewing the child individually in case she has any symptoms that she is hesitant to discuss in front of her parents. Children may not be comfortable revealing certain symptoms if they fear that their parents will disapprove or become upset with them. Accordingly, before proceeding with the assessment, the child and parents should agree on the extent to which symptom content will be shared with the parents. Depending on the nature of symptoms, it is also possible that youth may be fearful of saying their fears aloud. The other important factors to consider in the assessment of OCD are detailed below.

Family history

There is evidence that OCD is highly familial and has a genetic component. Thus, when considering a diagnosis of OCD, it may be helpful to inquire about family history of OCD or anxiety disorders, as this increases the likelihood of OCD. However, it is important to clarify that OCD is not the parents' or patient's fault, and that neither the child nor the parent(s) caused it.

Insight

Although many children and adolescents are aware of their OCD symptoms and the associated distress they experience as a result, other children may not have such awareness. Children may simply not recognize the bizarre, irrational, or excessive nature of their thoughts and behaviors. They may just feel that such behaviors are strong preferences (e.g., use of certain numbers). It may even seem as though children enjoy engaging in OCD-related behaviors. For instance, children may seek out compulsive behaviors (e.g., lining up toys) if they feel that those behaviors are rewarding or facilitate their playtime. Despite the potential lack of distress reported by the child, OCD symptoms frequently interfere with aspects of child and family functioning. Oftentimes, it is parents or caregivers who notice when such behaviors become excessive. In many instances though, the child is aware of the distressing nature of OCD and finds symptoms to be particularly overwhelming.

It is particularly important to assess a child's insight into the OCD, as this will likely impact the strategies used to get the child on board with OCD treatment. Since youth may not have good insight into symptoms, an initial assessment of OCD should include inquiring about the various common content areas of OCD obsessions and compulsions, as mentioned previously, as this may bring awareness of symptoms that the child engages in that may have otherwise gone undetected. Children may be suffering from symptoms of OCD but may not know that the symptoms are indicative of OCD and therefore may be treatable. Children may also have difficulty recognizing obsessions and the relationship between obsessions and compulsions. Treatment exercises may be used as an assessment tool to gain further assessment information. For instance, the child could be encouraged to participate in an exposure exercise to something that she avoids, and then when the child becomes distressed, the clinician could ask her what she is thinking.

Family accommodation

One of the most common methods by which OCD can affect the family is through family accommodation, which refers to how family members may participate in the obsessions and/or compulsions of a youth's OCD. Recognition of family accommodation is therefore important in assessing pediatric OCD. Family accommodation may consist of caregivers or siblings completing tasks for the youth with OCD because those activities are often associated with time-consuming rituals if she completes them independently. It may also consist of actual participation in the rituals to accommodate the youth (e.g., providing excessive reassurance to the youth with OCD), or modifying the family member's routine in an effort to avoid triggering the youth's OCD symptoms. Family members may become involved in the child's OCD to stop her from performing compulsions, to decrease the child's distress, or to hurry the child along when rituals are taking up excessive time. Youth may exhibit significant frustration or meltdowns if rituals are not accommodated. Parents often find themselves in a challenging position, as their child with OCD may struggle significantly to complete day-to-day tasks without assistance. Accordingly, family members may become involved in OCD symptoms, and this unfortunately only serves to maintain symptoms and reinforce the OCD because the youth does not gain practice with challenging symptoms independently.

Discriminating between OCD symptoms and normative development

It is important to differentiate symptoms of OCD from developmentally appropriate behaviors and behaviors that are normative in child development. The very task of identifying OCD can be challenging, as ritualistic and superstitious behaviors are normative to some extent in childhood. For instance, youth may have a bedtime routine, and this is not necessarily indicative of OCD. Children may insist on use of particular colors or numbers, or may request specific preparations for foods. One consideration is that rituals of children with OCD are typically associated with distress, whereas they are generally pleasurable in other children. Further, another distinguishing difference is whether impairment is associated with the behavior. Nonpathological superstitions and repetitive behaviors are not time consuming and do not result in clinically significant impairment or distress. Further, culturally prescribed ritual behavior is not itself indicative of OCD unless it exceeds cultural norms, occurs in situations judged as inappropriate by others of the same culture, and interferes with functioning.

Pediatric acute-onset neuropsychiatric syndrome (PANS)

This is a phenomenon characterized by a child exhibiting an abrupt and dramatic onset of OCD symptoms that is accompanied by the presence of additional neuropsychiatric symptoms, with similarly severe and acute onset, from at least two of the following seven categories:

1 anxiety

2 emotional liability and/or depression

3 irritability, aggression, and/or severely oppositional behaviors

4   behavioral (developmental) regression

5   sudden deterioration in school performance

6   sensory or motor abnormalities

7   somatic/physical signs and symptoms, including
    sleep disturbances, enuresis, or urinary frequency.

Additionally, symptoms cannot be better explained by a known neurologic or medical disorder. If such symptoms are observed in conjunction with the sudden onset of OCD symptoms, this classification of OCD should be considered.

Pediatric autoimmune neuropsychiatric disorders associated with streptococcus (PANDAS)

A possible association has also been shown in which patients develop OCD after experiencing a group A beta-hemolytic streptococcal infection. This subgroup of pediatric patients with OCD or tic disorders has been classified as PANDAS. In PANDAS, children show a rapid onset of significant behavioral changes and OCD symptoms temporally associated with a strep infection. All five of the following criteria must be met for PANDAS:

1   presence of obsessive compulsive disorder (OCD)
    or a tic disorder

2   prepubertal symptom onset

3   acute symptom onset and episodic
    (relapsing-remitting) course

4   temporal association between Group A
    streptococcal infection and symptom
    onset/exacerbations

5   associated with neurological abnormalities,
(particularly motoric hyperactivity and
choreiform movements).

If such symptoms occur in combination with the sudden
onset of OCD symptoms, this classification of OCD
should be considered.

Recognizing OCD at school

Given that children spend a significant portion of
their time in school, it is not surprising that OCD can
significantly impact school functioning and/or academic
performance. Thus, examination of school functioning
may be one means by which parents and professionals can
recognize OCD symptoms. A child with fears of germs or
contamination may make frequent trips to the bathroom to
wash her hands, excessively use hand sanitizer in the school
setting, or avoid touching shared school supplies. Youth
may excessively request to go to the school nurse, or may
excuse themselves to go to the bathroom frequently, due
to excessive concerns about illness or disease. Or, they may
avoid the school bathroom altogether if they have a fear of
public bathrooms. Children may feel the urge to go in and
out of doorways of classrooms or walk through hallways
in a particular way. Youth may feel the urge to save useless
items, such as scratch paper and/or wrappers, and they may
accumulate such items in their desk, backpack, or locker. Old
class notebooks may be saved in case they might be needed
sometime in the future. Organizing and arranging rituals
may also be observed by looking in a youth's backpack or on
her desk. Repetitive behaviors, such as reading paragraphs
over and over again, or erasing and re-writing are common

compulsions. Youth may also repetitively read instructions, check work to ensure accuracy, and/or seek reassurance from the teacher that a task has been completed accurately. Reassurance-seeking and/or confessing may also be present if the child is concerned about whether or not she broke school rules.

At school, OCD may also make it particularly challenging to concentrate. Children may be more concerned with obsessions and mental rituals than academic lessons, which may cause them to suffer academically, particularly if teachers are not understanding of such difficulties. One of the most common ways that OCD symptoms may interfere academically is through a child's engagement in mental rituals. Mental rituals may include behaviors such as counting behaviors or repeating certain phrases in one's mind. Mental rituals in OCD can seem similar to symptoms of other disorders (e.g., inattention present in attention deficit hyperactivity disorder), and therefore may not always be identified accurately. It may be particularly hard for a youth to concentrate on assignments or tests if she is experiencing intrusive thoughts or urges to complete mental rituals. OCD can also make children work in unproductive ways (e.g., re-writing letters to make them "just right"), which may be incorrectly perceived as noncompliance. Repetitive checking of work may interfere with timely completion of assignments and tests. Thus, the youth may experience negative academic consequences as a result of OCD symptoms. In severe circumstances, the child may regularly be absent from school due to the anxiety brought on by school-related triggers. There are also a variety of ways by which OCD can interfere with social functioning at school. A child may be hesitant to participate in physical education or sports due to contamination concerns related to touching equipment that is handled by other children. Rituals may also be particularly time consuming, which may preclude a youth from participating in extracurricular activities due to concerns that she will not have enough time to complete daily rituals. Youth with OCD may be teased if they engage in odd rituals or compulsions in the presence of peers. Overall, unexpected problems in academic or social functioning may be reason to suspect the presence of OCD symptoms. See Chapter 11 for a more thorough discussion of OCD in the school setting.

Examining the role of thinking in OCD

A useful method of recognizing OCD can be through the identification of thought patterns common in OCD. Most individuals experience intrusive thoughts that are similar in subject matter to the obsessions found in OCD, yet these thoughts appear to differ from OCD thoughts in several ways. Compared to obsessions, normal unwanted thoughts occur less frequently, are interpreted differently, are less intense, are more controllable, and are less likely to be associated with ritualizing. Cognitive–behavioral models of OCD suggest that dysfunctional beliefs and interpretations of normally occurring intrusive thoughts generate the highly distressing and time-consuming obsessions and compulsions. This is thought to occur when the intrusions are considered to be highly important and as posing a threat for which the individual with OCD is personally responsible. Thus, biases in thinking may help differentiate obsessions versus normal intrusive thoughts. Accordingly, identification of these inaccurate beliefs may be helpful in recognizing symptoms as OCD.

Some of these thinking traps may include excessive doubting, intolerance of uncertainty, overestimating probability, catastrophic thinking, an inflated sense of responsibility, over-importance of thoughts, and thought–action fusion, which we now discuss. Children with OCD may often experience excessive doubting. Youth may report excessive doubts regarding whether or not they performed certain actions (e.g., "I can't remember if I checked the door lock"). Further, those with OCD tend to have less confidence in their memories, and this uncertainty causes them to engage in compulsive behaviors. Intolerance of uncertainty is another cognitive trap often identified in OCD. Those with OCD may experience beliefs that it is necessary to be 100 percent certain. Any hint of doubt or ambiguity is perceived as unacceptable. Accordingly, they may engage in compulsive behaviors in order to achieve an increased sense of control instead of tolerating uncertainty. Overestimating probability is also commonly seen in OCD and reflects an exaggeration of the probability of harm or another negative outcome. Outcomes that have a low likelihood of occurring are erroneously perceived to have a higher likelihood of occurring ("The chances of contracting HIV if I use a public bathroom is at least 20 percent"). Or, individuals may exaggerate the seriousness of any negative consequences. Catastrophic thinking occurs when one automatically thinks that the worst-case scenario has or will occur despite the lack of evidence ("I'll get sick and die if I go near sick people without washing afterwards").

Inflated responsibility is the erroneous belief that one has the special power to cause, and/or the duty to prevent, negative outcomes. Intrusive thoughts are interpreted as having implications for taking action to prevent harm, and the child with OCD would feel that the neglect of taking action would in turn imply blame. Consequently, the child will engage in corrective or preventative action in order to alleviate the distress associated with her feelings of inflated responsibility. An example might be that a child with OCD feels that she has to say a special phrase or prayer before her parent leaves the home to prevent a car accident from occurring. A thinking error related to inflated responsibility is over-importance of thoughts, which is the belief that the presence of a thought indicates that it must be important (e.g., "Having an unwanted thought of committing harm must mean I really want to do it"). Within this domain is thought-action fusion. Thought-action fusion (TAF) is a distorted way of thinking that often presents in two forms: "probability TAF" is when the intrusive thought itself is believed to increase the probability that a specific negative event will occur, such as "If I think about falling ill, it makes it more likely that I will become ill." "Morality TAF" is when experiencing the intrusive thought is believed to be morally equivalent to carrying out a prohibited action, such as "If I think about swearing in church, this is almost as bad as actually swearing in church." TAF is currently viewed as one of a number of ways in which too much significance is placed on the meaning of their thoughts by people with obsessional difficulties. Studies also show that TAF triggers efforts to neutralize or suppress thoughts, which counterproductively increases obsessive compulsive symptoms.

As a result of learning to identify these patterns of thinking, parents and children have a tool that will help in combating OCD. If symptoms can be appropriately labeled as OCD, it is more likely that they will apply treatment strategies to the symptoms. Cognitive restructuring is used throughout treatment to help the child evaluate perceived threats associated with obsessions more appropriately (e.g., how likely is it that you'll actually become sick after shaking someone's hands?). This also allows the youth to test hypotheses based on the beliefs about the perceived threat. Individuals are taught to evaluate the accuracy of their thoughts through use of Socratic questioning, or as a result of behavioral experiments to test whether the feared outcome actually comes true.

Differential diagnosis

There are many psychological disorders that have characteristics similar to those displayed by individuals with OCD. Accordingly, separating OCD from other conditions can be challenging due to the similar expressions of some symptoms. It is important to note that for an accurate diagnosis of OCD, the obsessions and compulsions should not be better explained by other disorders. Overall, it is important to make sure symptoms are accurately identified as OCD to guide appropriate treatment planning and intervention.

Generalized anxiety disorder (GAD)

GAD is characterized by excessive and hard to control anxiety and worry about a number of events or activities. The pervasive worries present in GAD can seem similar to obsessions in OCD, as both represent excessive and/or uncontrollable cognitive processes associated with negative affect (Brown *et al.* 1993). In GAD, worries are considered reflective of real-life circumstances and everyday concerns, such as academics, health, interpersonal relationships, family, finances, and news, yet are clearly excessive.

However, in OCD, worries are more likely to have an irrational or bizarre nature. The DSM specifies that obsessions in OCD are not simply excessive worries about real-life problems. The content of obsessions in OCD tend to be experienced as contradictory to one's own beliefs and values, whereas worries in GAD tend to be experienced as more consistent with one's own beliefs and values. A diagnosis of GAD also specifies that a child must exhibit at least one physical symptom associated with worry, whereas this criterion is not specified in OCD. However, this factor alone cannot serve to differentiate GAD versus OCD as physical/somatic symptoms are also often present in OCD. OCD is also typically characterized by the key feature of overt compulsions, which can facilitate differential diagnosis (Brown *et al.* 1993).

Specific phobias

Specific phobias are characterized by marked and persistent fear that is excessive or unreasonable, cued by the presence or anticipation of a specific object, animal, or situation. Individuals with OCD may similarly fear objects, situations, or events. Further, avoidance of the thing that causes their fear is common among people with both OCD and specific phobias. In OCD, the fear and avoidance of a specific object or situation is related to avoiding the triggering of an obsession or compulsion (e.g., avoidance of dirt due to a contamination obsession). However, the fears in specific phobia do not linger as much when the feared stimuli are not near. In OCD, the individual will obsess about the fear outside of the feared situation or event. Unlike a specific phobia of a disease or illness, which generally entails a fear of *contracting* an illness, OCD concerns related to illness are typically associated with a conviction that one *already has* a serious illness. OCD can also be differentiated from a specific phobia of illness due to the presence of compulsions. Individuals with specific phobias do not usually adopt compulsive behaviors to relieve their anxiety. For example, when a fear of vomiting occurs in the context of OCD, there are generally extensive rituals (e.g., compulsive hand washing, checking expiration dates) to reduce/avoid the risk of vomiting, even in the absence of a trigger.

Social phobia

Social phobia is distinguished by a marked and persistent fear of one or more social situations. The individual fears that she will act in a way that will be humiliating or embarrassing. Accordingly, the feared social situations are either avoided or endured with intense anxiety or distress. Thus, the differential diagnosis of social phobia over OCD is first based on whether the fear is primarily social, as in social phobia fears are particularly limited to social situations. Nonetheless, avoidance of social situations may be indicated in OCD as well. OCD is often associated with avoidance of situations that are the focus of obsessions, and such situations may overlap with commonly avoided situations in social phobia. Youth with OCD may fear being around others due to contamination concerns or a fear of not saying the right thing. Youth with a fear of germs may avoid public bathrooms or eating at restaurants. To determine differential diagnosis, it is necessary to determine the reason for the avoidance. A person with social phobia will avoid such situations because of concerns about negative evaluations by others, whereas an individual with OCD would avoid such situations due to concerns about contamination resulting from public contact. If an individual with OCD avoids social situations only because of concerns that others will notice her excessive hand washing, a diagnosis of social phobia would not be assigned. Correct differential diagnosis therefore depends on the focus of the individual's anxiety, reasons for avoidance, and range of situations feared. OCD and social phobia may both involve reassurance-seeking behavior, but in social phobia such reassurance-seeking is focused on reducing the social fears.

Separation anxiety disorder

Separation anxiety disorder is described as developmentally inappropriate or excessive anxiety regarding separation from those to whom the child is attached. The underlying fear is losing or becoming separated from caregivers. One of the most common overlapping fears in OCD and separation anxiety is a fear of possible harm befalling caregivers. In OCD, the youth may feel the need to engage in compulsive behaviors in an effort to prevent something bad from happening to caregivers. Youth may engage in bizarre and unrelated behaviors, such as saying a particular phrase or doing something until it feels "right," to prevent harm to caregivers. In separation anxiety, associated behaviors typically include reluctance to be without attachment figures due to fears. Further, in separation anxiety, the youth may experience repeated nightmares involving the theme of separation, whereas that is less common in youth with OCD.

Post-traumatic stress disorder (PTSD)

Both OCD and PTSD may be associated with unpleasant thoughts or images that are distressing and difficult to control. The content of the thoughts and images present in PTSD is typically associated with re-experiencing a trauma. However, it is possible for individuals with OCD to experience intrusive images associated with a prior adverse event. In PTSD, individuals must exhibit at least two symptoms of increased arousal. Both PTSD and OCD may be associated with uncomfortable physical symptoms. The role of physical symptoms in OCD is hard to parse out as somatic concerns also characterize the nature of some children's obsessions and/or compulsions. Examining the role of physical symptoms in OCD may be challenging as it may be difficult to differentiate between a child's actual experience of somatic complaints and preoccupation with such concerns. Gathering information about the situations that typically surround the onset of physical symptoms is likely to be more helpful in determining a diagnosis than solely assessing the presence of a particular somatic complaint.

Hypochondriasis

In hypochondriasis, individuals fear that they have contracted an illness or disease, or fear that something is seriously wrong with their health. In OCD, most of the concerns include worries about becoming ill or contracting a disease in the future. Thus, a child will engage in significant efforts to decrease the likelihood of becoming ill in the future. The DSM provides guidance by indicating that if the distressing thoughts are exclusively related to fears of having, or the idea that one has, a serious disease based on misinterpretation of bodily symptoms, then hypochondriasis should be diagnosed instead of OCD.

Body dysmorphic disorder (BDD)

BDD is closely related to OCD, and is characterized by preoccupation with imagined or slight defects in appearance. If a slight anomaly is present, the person's concern may be excessive. The preoccupation causes distress and impairment in functioning. Common preoccupations focus on the skin (e.g., acne), hair (e.g., baldness, excessive facial or body hair), or nose (e.g., size, shape), although any body part could be the focus of concern. Most individuals with BDD perform specific behaviors, such as mirror checking and skin-picking, which are linked to preoccupation with their appearance. Other common behaviors can include excessive grooming, washing one's face excessively, reassurance-seeking, excessive exercise, and avoidance of social situations due to fears that they will be judged by others as "ugly." Checking rituals are common in BDD but tend to be restricted to behaviors related to the perceived defect, such as repetitive examinations of one's face. If preoccupations and repetitive behaviors focus on appearance, BDD should likely be diagnosed rather than OCD. Level of insight may also inform differential diagnosis, as studies consistently show that insight in BDD tends to be poorer than in OCD.

Hoarding disorder

Hoarding disorder is characterized by persistent difficulty getting rid of possessions, regardless of their value. Symptoms may include thoughts of needing to save or keep things that others would likely throw away (e.g., trash, wrappers, ribbons, string), and excessive concern with discarding items of sentimental value (e.g., old toys). Oftentimes, this results in excessive clutter of unnecessary items in one's environment. Youth may also save needless paperwork or notes/assignments from previous school years due to concerns that they may need those items later. If excessive items are saved in OCD, it is usually due to the presence of obsessions or compulsions (e.g., needing to check items before they are discarded). Accordingly, hoarding disorder is not diagnosed if the symptoms are determined to be a direct consequence of obsessions or compulsions.

Attention deficit hyperactivity disorder (ADHD)

Depending on type, ADHD may be characterized by inattention, hyperactivity, and/or impulsivity. Given that OCD can be associated with significant preoccupation with obsessions and/or the presence of mental rituals, OCD symptoms may be misconstrued as symptoms of inattention or distractibility. What may appear as distractibility in ADHD may actually be the performance of mental rituals, which are often present in OCD. A child with OCD may have difficulty progressing through an assignment due to re-reading or re-writing behaviors. It is important to ensure that the attention problems resultant from preoccupation with obsessions and compulsions are not incorrectly labeled as ADHD. Children with OCD may display attentional abnormalities and impulsive behaviors that are not best attributed to ADHD. Thus, a very careful assessment into the nature and presentation of such symptoms is imperative prior to making a diagnosis.

Depression

In depression, individuals may experience depressive ruminations that seem similar to the obsessions and intrusive thoughts often present in OCD. However, in depression, ruminations are typically about pessimistic ideas about the self or the world. In OCD, there are more attempts to suppress thoughts, unlike in depression. Rumination in depression is also more past oriented, whereas rumination in OCD may be more related to how symptoms will impact the future (e.g., future-oriented worry). Depression may be characterized by recurrent ruminations that are usually mood congruent and not necessarily experienced as intrusive or distressing. The DSM discusses that a depressed individual who ruminates that she is worthless would not be considered to have obsessions because such behavior is not ego dystonic. Depressive ruminations are not linked to compulsions, as is typical of OCD.

Autism spectrum disorders (ASD)

Individuals with ASD often have restrictive and stereotyped behaviors, activities, or interests (APA 2013). They may be inflexible to changes in routine and may display rigidity with their schedule, so disruptions to the routine will typically cause significant distress due to rigidity and inflexibility with change. The outward presentation of obsessions and compulsions in OCD, and fixated interests and repetitive behaviors in ASD, may pose a challenge when attempting to make an accurate diagnosis due to their similar phenotypic presentations.

Obsessions in OCD are typically considered as ego dystonic, meaning that they are contrary to the individual's self-concept and belief system. Accordingly, they are considered intrusive and distressing, and they do not provide pleasure or gratification. Contrarily, individuals with ASD with fixated interests often get pleasure from the content of the repetitive thoughts and they might get enjoyment from focusing on a particular topic. Further, those with ASD may possess restricted interests and have difficulty diverging from their fixated interest during play or in conversations with others.

Due to difficulty distinguishing OCD and ASD based on their outward presentations, it can be helpful to examine what purpose the behavior serves for the individual as well as the context the behavior occurs in. Repetitive behaviors in OCD typically reduce distress or anxiety, whereas repetitive behaviors in ASD may serve as self-soothing or self-stimulatory behaviors. In OCD, a repetitive behavior might be exhibited with the intent to counteract thoughts about something catastrophic happening if the repetitive behavior is not completed. Individuals with ASD may engage in the same behavior as a way of self-soothing, and the behavior is not exhibited to attenuate anxiety or prevent a feared outcome. In ASD, routines or repetitive behaviors are typically driven by rigidity, whereas in OCD they are more driven by fears of doing something wrong or something bad happening rather than simply rigidity. In OCD, compulsions serve as a way to avoid undesired stimuli, negatively reinforcing the compulsions. In ASD, the behaviors are self-soothing or provide a sense of comfort, positively reinforcing these behaviors. The reasons behind the behaviors are typically different and thus are important to consider in the assessment process.

When seeking differential diagnosis of OCD and ASD, it may also be helpful to examine clinical presentations of ASD outside of the symptom overlap. In distinguishing

ASD from OCD, it may be particularly helpful to focus on social functioning and behavior. Individuals with ASD often exhibit difficulty with social relationships and lack reciprocal social interaction skills. Assessment of language or other developmental delays may also be helpful in differentiating ASD from OCD, as individuals with ASD are often delayed in language development. Children with ASD may have preoccupations with unusual objects or parts of objects, yet are typically less bothered by these preoccupations than those that are present in OCD. Individuals with ASD may engage in self-stimulatory behaviors or stereotypes such as hand flapping or body rocking.

Tics

A tic is a sudden, rapid, recurrent, nonrhythmic, stereotyped motor movement or vocalization. Tics often closely resemble the repetitive or ritualistic behavior exhibited by those with OCD. In distinguishing between OCD compulsions and tics, it may be helpful to assess what precedes the behavior along with evaluating the function served by the behavior. Tics are more likely to be associated with premonitory urges just prior to the behavior. Premonitory urges are typically characterized by physical tension or sensory discomfort in particular locations of the body. Premonitory urges can be likened to the need to sneeze or to scratch an itch. The performance of the tic itself is usually associated with a feeling of relief from this uncomfortable urge or physical tension. An OCD compulsion is more likely to be preceded by cognitive content in the form of fears or obsessions. Such cognitive content is typically accompanied by affective arousal states (e.g., anxiety, distress), which are typically reduced upon performance of compulsions.

Accordingly, compulsions are performed to reduce anxiety associated with obsessions. Whereas obsessions are typically associated with feelings of anxiety or distress, premonitory urges are less likely to directly produce anxiety. Tics are less complex than compulsions and are not aimed at neutralizing obsessions. A useful question in assessment may therefore be whether withholding of the behavior results in anxiety versus sensory discomfort. Given that obsessions are more likely associated with specific fears than premonitory urges, it can be helpful to assess whether the youth thinks that any feared events may occur if she were to withhold the behavior. Responses such as "something bad might happen" may be more indicative of OCD phenomenology, whereas responses such as "I can't hold it in" or "the urge would just get stronger" are more indicative of tic disorder phenomenology.

Simple tics can usually be identified based on their quick duration, simplicity of movement, lack of purposefulness, and perceived involuntariness. Complex and seemingly ritualistic tics typically follow the onset of simple tics and are rarely the only tics present. Accordingly, if complex tics seem to be the only symptom, the behaviors may be better conceptualized as compulsions. If the child exhibits only brief and meaningless repetitive behaviors in the absence of any cognitive or affective precursors, a tic disorder may be a more appropriate diagnosis. Further, tics are generally experienced as less voluntary than compulsions.

Disruptive behavior

It may be challenging to differentiate OCD and oppositional/defiant behavior, as the rigidity of compulsive behavior can mimic oppositional behavior in children.

In OCD, the child may report distressing and intrusive violent thoughts that are not aligned with her own reported wishes. To differentiate whether symptoms are due to OCD or actual aggressive intentions, it is important to establish whether the violent thoughts and images are unwanted. If the child is excited by the violent thoughts/images or expresses an intention toward following through with the thoughts, OCD may be ruled out. It is also important to differentiate normative, ego-syntonic thoughts that occur in the context of anger (e.g., "I'd just like to hit her since she broke my Barbie") from symptoms better classified as OCD.

Parents and professionals should also work to differentiate problem behaviors arising as a result of OCD and problem behaviors stemming from oppositionality. An important consideration is whether the child receives any secondary gain (e.g., getting out of chores) as a result of reported symptoms. Secondary gain may occur in an effort to prevent distress in the child with OCD. Family accommodation of the child's OCD often results in secondary gain (e.g., greater attention, different expectations than other children).

Psychosis

Individuals with OCD recognize that the obsessions are a product of one's own mind and are not imposed from without (as in thought insertion). The DSM discusses that the ruminative delusional thoughts and bizarre stereotyped behaviors in schizophrenia are differentiated from obsessions and compulsions by the fact that they are not ego dystonic and not subject to reality testing. People with paranoia and psychosis are more likely to believe that the causes of their fears are real and that their fears are rational, whereas most individuals with OCD recognize that symptoms are excessive and irrational. When conducting an assessment, questions should differentiate between voices (as in psychosis) and intrusive thoughts (as in OCD). In psychosis, recurrent thoughts are held with delusional conviction. Such delusional thoughts might also be accompanied by other characteristic symptoms of schizophrenia (e.g., hallucinations, disorganized speech, negative symptoms).

Anorexia nervosa

Individuals with anorexia nervosa often exhibit a significant fear of gaining weight or becoming fat, and they often experience a preoccupation with their body weight or shape. Further, there is often a preoccupation with thoughts of food. Although obsessive compulsive features may seem present, a primary distinguishing factor between anorexia nervosa and OCD is that in OCD, the obsessions and compulsions are not limited to concerns about weight and food.

Conclusion

This chapter sought to provide guidance for children, parents, and professionals in recognizing OCD. Common themes in pediatric OCD were reviewed, as well as a variety of factors to consider in the assessment process. It also discussed how completing an accurate differential diagnosis can prove challenging due to the similar phenotypic expressions of symptoms in different psychological disorders. However, accurately attributing the symptoms to the appropriate disorder will allow for the proper intervention. Unfortunately, many youth with OCD go undiagnosed or misdiagnosed, which likely contributes to significant impairment and maintenance of symptoms. Thus, improvement in the assessment and recognition of OCD is an important area of focus.

5

NOW WHAT?

SELECTING THE RIGHT OBSESSIVE COMPULSIVE DISORDER TREATMENT FOR CHILDREN AND ADOLESCENTS

Joseph F. McGuire

Introduction

As obsessive compulsive disorder (OCD) does not get better without treatment, pursuing the right treatment in a timely fashion is important. The first step is a comprehensive clinical assessment, which is used to accurately determine diagnoses, symptom severity, and the level of family accommodation. The use of evidence-based rating scales across assessment and treatment is helpful to objectively evaluate symptom severity and monitor responsiveness to treatment. When reviewing the literature, there are two well-studied treatments that are effective for childhood OCD. These are cognitive-behavioral therapy (CBT) and a group of medications called serotonin reuptake inhibitors (SRIs). In medical research, randomized controlled trials (RCTs) are the "gold standard" measure to evaluate the benefit of a treatment. Both qualitative literature reviews (Franklin *et al.* 2015) and quantitative evaluations of RCTs (McGuire *et al.* 2015) have found considerable empirical support for both CBT and SRI treatments relative to comparison conditions. This chapter provides a brief introduction to the treatment of childhood OCD with CBT and SSRI medications, and provides recommendations for treatment based on available empirical evidence.

What is cognitive behavioral therapy?

There are many different types of psychotherapy, and not all are appropriate for the treatment of childhood OCD. Cognitive behavioral therapy (CBT) is a specific type of psychotherapy that focuses on the interaction between thoughts, behaviors, and feelings. It is goal oriented and time limited. Although the cognitive-behavioral model of OCD is discussed more fully in another chapter, briefly this model suggests that patients with OCD experience repetitive distressing thoughts called *obsessions*. In an attempt to reduce distress from obsessive thoughts, those with OCD engage in ritualistic behaviors that serve to temporarily reduce distress. These are called *compulsions*. Patients may actively avoid obsession-related triggers to minimize daily distress, which serves a similar function as compulsions. This is called *avoidance*. Patients with OCD become increasingly reliant on ritualized behaviors or avoidance strategies to cope with obsession-induced distress. In addition to being maladaptive, dependence on ritualized and/or avoidant behaviors prohibits new learning from taking place that could help patients recognize that these behaviors are not necessary to prevent feared outcomes and/or reduce distress. In CBT, patients learn to face the fear and distress associated with obsessions through repeated practice exercises called *exposures*. As patients practice facing their fears in a gradual manner while refraining from engaging in compulsive behaviors, they habituate to the fear and distress triggered by obsessions and learn that feared outcomes are unrealistic and compulsions are not needed. Specific examples of OCD symptoms and their treatment with exposures in CBT can be found in Chapters 4 and 7.

Components of CBT

Evidence-based CBT for childhood OCD includes multiple therapeutic components. The common core components across standardized CBT treatments include psychoeducation about OCD, symptom hierarchy development, cognitive strategies, and exposure and response prevention (ERP). Psychoeducation is a central component of CBT for any psychiatric condition. It provides patients and parents with information about OCD, discusses the cognitive-behavioral model of OCD, and orients patients and parents to the procedures involved in treatment. In symptom hierarchy development, the CBT clinician, patient, and/or parents collaboratively construct a treatment hierarchy consisting of the patient's obsessive compulsive symptoms (e.g., obsessive thoughts, compulsive rituals, avoidance behaviors). The construction of a symptom hierarchy allows for treatment to initially focus on symptoms that evoke less fear and/or distress to start. As patients develop mastery over these initial exercises, they progress through the treatment hierarchy to master more challenging/distressing exposures. Cognitive training is another component of evidence-based CBT that varies according to the patient's developmental level, cognitive functioning, and insight into OCD symptoms. Typically, cognitive strategies focus on reducing externalizing OCD symptoms (i.e., as a common adversary against whom the patient, parent and clinician will ally in order to combat), practicing constructive self-talk (e.g., "I'm going to beat OCD"), and engaging in cognitive restructuring. These components are integral to the goal of providing tools for later use in exposure activities (e.g., helping patients view exposures as "an opportunity to fight OCD"). In ERP, the patient repeatedly confronts symptoms on their treatment hierarchy through exposure exercises and practice resisting engagement in compulsive behaviors. Through these exposures, patients habituate to the distress triggered by obsessions and learn that compulsive behaviors (or avoidance) are not needed to reduce distress. Furthermore, patients learn that previously feared outcomes are inaccurate and/or unlikely. As patients practice exposures, the frequency and intensity of OCD symptom severity decreases.

Along with these core CBT components, there are two specific aspects of CBT of childhood OCD worth touching upon. First, as youth with OCD may initially resist participation in treatment, the incorporation of a reward-based system to motivate patients to engage in therapy sessions and later exposure activities is important. The reward-based system should be developmentally appropriate and collaboratively developed between patients and parents. Token economy reward-based systems are often used in treatment and can be modified across the developmental spectrum to encourage therapy session participation as well as compliance with exposures outside of session (called homework). Practicing CBT tasks outside of visits with your therapist is an integral aspect of positive therapeutic outcomes in childhood OCD.

Second, as family accommodation is often present in childhood OCD, family involvement in treatment is strongly encouraged. Parental involvement can help reduce family accommodation in a gradual manner and facilitate structured implementation of treatment outside of the CBT sessions by helping children complete exposures. Moreover, parents often benefit from observing clinician-guided exposures that utilize non-coercive and supportive techniques to help patients overcome their symptoms. These clinician-guided exposures can help parents and/or family members reduce blaming, reprimanding, and/or accommodating that can occur when confronting OCD symptoms outside of therapy.

Empirical evidence for CBT

There is considerable empirical support for CBT in the treatment of OCD in children and adolescents. There have been many RCTs evaluating the benefit of structured CBT protocols for youth with OCD. These trials have compared CBT to multiple different types of comparison conditions (e.g., waitlists, placebo pill, treatment-as-usual, relaxation training) and found CBT to be significantly superior (McGuire *et al.* 2015). In medical research, the benefit of treatment relative to comparison conditions is quantified using a measure called an effect size; the bigger the effect size, the larger the treatment gains (small effect size: 0.00–0.50; medium effect size: 0.50–0.80; large effect size: 0.80–2.0). Across these RCTs, CBT was associated with a very large treatment effect size (1.21) (McGuire *et al.* 2015). Furthermore, up to 80 percent of patients exhibited a treatment response to CBT, with as many as 57 percent of patients experiencing diagnostic remission (McGuire *et al.* 2015). Treatment gains from CBT have been maintained for up to seven years after initial treatment (O'Leary, Barrett, and Fjermestad 2009).

Research has identified several factors associated with CBT treatment response among youth with OCD. Positive treatment effects of CBT have been associated with more therapeutic contact and homework compliance. Meanwhile, factors associated with a diminished treatment response to CBT include greater OCD symptom severity, the presence of specific co-occurring psychiatric conditions (e.g., attention deficit hyperactivity disorder (ADHD), depression, or disruptive behaviors), poor insight into OCD symptoms, prominent hoarding symptoms, and greater levels of family accommodation. These factors can impede CBT and should be taken into consideration by the treatment team. Additionally, it is important to clarify that a diminished treatment response does not mean that CBT does not provide any therapeutic benefit. Rather, youth who have factors associated with a diminished treatment response may require more intensive treatment, longer duration of treatment, and/or other modifications from standardized treatment protocols used in these RCTs.

Duration and course of CBT treatment

The structured CBT protocols used in RCTs typically consist of 12 to 14 hour-long weekly therapy sessions. However, in clinical practice, the number of CBT sessions can vary considerably based on a patient's OCD symptom severity, progress in treatment, and scheduling constraints. For instance, an older adolescent patient with good insight into his OCD symptoms and who completes out-of-session exposures regularly may require fewer treatment sessions, whereas a younger patient with poor insight into his symptoms and with lower homework compliance may require more CBT sessions. As patients improve over the course of CBT, weekly sessions may be tapered to biweekly or monthly meetings to provide patients and families with a gradual transition of supportive therapeutic discontinuation. Although weekly sessions are the standard of care for CBT, intensive CBT approaches that consist of daily sessions have also demonstrated significant benefit for patients with severe OCD when conducted over one to three weeks. While these intensive therapeutic approaches can be offered in an outpatient format, they are more readily found in the context of partial hospitalization programs or residential treatment facilities.

What are SRI medications?

There are many different types of medications that have been evaluated in the treatment of OCD in children and adolescents. SRIs are a group of medications that include clomipramine (trade name Anafranil) and more selective serotonin reuptake inhibitors (SSRIs) such as sertraline (trade name Zoloft), fluoxetine (trade name Prozac), paroxetine (trade name Paxil), and fluvoxamine (trade name Luvox). These five SRI medications have been approved by the United States Food and Drug Administration (FDA) for the treatment of OCD. While citalopram (trade name Celexa) and escitalopram (trade name Lexapro) are both medications that influence serotonin reuptake, they have not been rigorously tested among children and adolescents with OCD in RCTs. Although neurobiological models of OCD are discussed more fully in a later chapter, briefly these medications reduce OCD symptoms by increasing the amount of the neurotransmitter called serotonin in synapses throughout the brain. While the benefits of SRI medications initially implicated a serotonin deficit among patients with OCD, further research suggests there to be multiple underlying causes of OCD.

Components of pharmacologic treatment

There are multiple components to the pharmacologic treatment of childhood OCD. Core components include psychoeducation, symptom assessment and monitoring, medication prescription/titration, and side effect monitoring. Psychoeducation for medication management provides patients and parents with information about OCD and orients them to procedures involved in treatment. Psychoeducation in the context of pharmacotherapy focuses on the neurobiological model of OCD and describes how SRI medications can improve OCD symptoms. In symptom assessment and monitoring, the presence and severity of the patient's OCD symptoms are assessed. The gold standard assessment measure used in RCTs is a semi-structured interview called the Children's Yale-Brown Obsessive Compulsive Scale (Scahill *et al.* 1997). As structured interviews often take considerable time to administer, clinicians may also rely upon parent and/or child report measures of OCD symptom severity. Medication management includes selecting an evidence-based medication, titrating the medication to an optimal dose, and monitoring for medication side effects. Some common side effects of SRI medications include insomnia, nausea, gastrointestinal problems, sexual problems, dizziness, and sedation. In addition to these common side effects, clomipramine has been reported to be accompanied by weight gain and anticholinergic side effects. While side effects typically emerge during the initial treatment phase, evidence suggests that side effects subside in many cases as treatment continues. Although infrequently occurring, there are two serious side effects associated with SRI medications: behavioral activation and increased suicidality. Behavioral activation is characterized by a variety of symptoms such as agitation, aggression, irritability, impulsivity, and increased anxiety or depression. Meanwhile, increased suicidality is characterized by an increase in suicidal thoughts and behaviors—but not necessarily suicide attempts. Because increased suicidality occurs in a small fraction of youth on SRI medications, it has resulted in an FDA black box warning. While these side effect profiles can be concerning, multiple RCTs provide evidence that the benefits of using SRIs to treatment childhood OCD generally outweighs the possible risks, which can be reduced with careful monitoring.

Empirical evidence for SRI medications

There is considerable empirical support for SRI medications for the treatment of OCD in children and adolescents. Generally, RCTs have typically compared SRI medications to placebos over a course of eight to 16 weeks, and found SRI medications to be significantly more effective (Geller *et al.* 2003b; McGuire *et al.* 2015). Across RCTs, SRI medications were associated with a moderate treatment effect size (0.50) (McGuire *et al.* 2015). Furthermore, up to 50 percent of patients exhibited a positive treatment response, but rates of remission are lower, ranging from 21 to 47 percent (McGuire *et al.* 2015). While treatment gains from SRI medications can persist after medication discontinuation, some youth experience a return of OCD symptoms when the SRI medication is withdrawn. When comparing SRI medications to one another, no single SRI medication appears to be consistently superior in reducing OCD symptom severity. However, a quantitative summary of RCTs that examined the therapeutic benefit across trials found some evidence that clomipramine may be superior to other SRI medications (Geller *et al.* 2003b).

Although no specific factors have been associated with a positive treatment response to SRI medications, a few factors have been found to be associated with a diminished treatment response. These factors predominantly focus on the presence of co-occurring psychiatric conditions like ADHD, oppositional defiance disorder (ODD), predominant hoarding symptoms, and tics/tic disorders (Geller *et al.* 2003a; March *et al.* 2007). Notably, a diminished treatment response does not mean that the patient does not experience any benefit from the medication. Rather, the reduction in OCD symptom severity experienced may not be clinically significant for the dose and duration used in the RCTs when these conditions are present. Furthermore, clinical evidence suggests that a patient's poor response to one SRI medication is not indicative of his response to other SRI medications. Indeed, expert clinical guidelines recommend an adequate trial of three or more SRI medications before considering a patient to be unresponsive.

Duration and course of pharmacotherapy

The frequency and duration of medication management appointments vary over the course of treatment. Initial visits may occur more often and last longer while SRI medications are being titrated and side effects closely monitored. Once an optimum therapeutic dose is achieved with minimal side effects, medication management sessions may occur less frequently. Experts generally recommend that SRI medications be tried for at least 12 weeks at an adequate dose before switching to another SRI medication is considered.

The FDA-recommended target doses for SRIs in childhood OCD are sertraline (100 to 200 mg), fluoxetine (20 to 60 mg), fluvoxamine (100 to 300 mg), and paroxetine (20 to 60 mg). Once an optimal therapeutic dose is achieved, expert guidelines recommend the continuation of SRI medications for at least one year. Depending on the patient's clinical presentation and possible side effect profile after a year, SRI discontinuation may be considered and should be collaboratively discussed between patients, parents, and the treating clinician.

CBT and SRI medications: comparisons and combined treatment

When comparing CBT and SRI medications to one another, CBT was found to reduce OCD symptom severity better than SRI medications across all studies. While the small number of childhood OCD studies needs to be considered, CBT was reported to be the preferred treatment option for parents of youth with OCD when compared to SRI medications or the combined treatment (CBT + an SRI medication; Lewin *et al.* 2014).

While CBT and SRI medications are beneficial by themselves, the combination of these two therapies is a strong treatment for childhood OCD. The implementation of this combined treatment typically takes one of three approaches. First, CBT and a SRI medication are initiated at the same time. In a large-scale RCT, this treatment approach was associated with a large treatment effect (1.4), with up to 53 percent of patients experiencing diagnostic remission (POTS 2004). Despite these robust findings, no significant difference has been found between children who receive CBT+ an SRI medication compared to CBT alone (POTS 2004; Storch *et al.* 2013). Second, SRI medications are initiated first with CBT incorporated into treatment afterward. A large RCT used this treatment approach and found that the addition of CBT to ongoing SRI treatment was superior to ongoing SRI treatment alone (Franklin *et al.* 2015). This treatment approach was associated with a large treatment effect (0.85), with up to 69 percent of patients experiencing a treatment response after CBT was incorporated into treatment. The third approach involves youth being unresponsive to a standard course of CBT and subsequently adding an SRI medication to improve therapeutic response. A large-scale RCT examined whether patients with OCD who did not exhibit a significant improvement after 14 weekly CBT sessions improved better with the addition of an SRI medication or with ongoing CBT sessions (Skarphedinsson *et al.* 2015). The addition of an SRI medication was associated with a large treatment effect (1.19), with up to 45 percent of patients experiencing a treatment response after 16 weeks of SRI treatment. Meanwhile, the continuation of CBT sessions for an additional 16 weeks was associated with a large treatment effect (1.04), with up to 50 percent of patients experiencing a treatment response.

Which is the best treatment option?

The timely decision to pursue treatment for childhood OCD is important. Multiple factors can influence treatment decisions such as a patient's OCD severity, access to therapeutic services, patient/family preferences, side effect profiles, and responsiveness to treatment. Based on available scientific evidence, expert guidelines recommend CBT as the initial treatment choice for children and adolescents with mild-to-moderate OCD symptom severity or when co-occurring tics are present (Bloch and Storch 2015; Geller and March 2012). While many patients with mild-to-moderate severity will respond to a standard course of CBT, some may not experience a significant benefit due to several possible factors (e.g., minimal CBT homework compliance). For these patients who do not respond to a standard course of CBT, the addition of an SRI medication or continued CBT can provide additional therapeutic benefit. As patients may not initially respond to the first SRI medication, other SRI medications should be evaluated after an adequate trial of the first SRI medication is complete. Once an optimal SRI medication and dose are identified, the SRI medication should be maintained for at least one year with the CBT sessions tapered down slowly.

For youth with mild-to-moderate OCD severity who do not have immediate access to CBT or for patients who are unwilling to initially participate in CBT, SRI medications can be used as an initial treatment step. SRI medication selection may likely occur based on the patient's medical history, possible medication interactions with existing medications, and potential side effects associated with each specific SRI medication. For example, a specific SRI medication may be preferred because it has few negative interactions with medications prescribed for the patient's other medical conditions, or because its common side effect profile (e.g., sedation, tiredness) may be less aversive than others (e.g., gastrointestinal issues). Similarly, while some evidence may suggest that clomipramine may be more beneficial medication, it requires close side effect monitoring in case of rare but serious adverse effects (e.g., seizures, electrocardiogram changes). Given the complexities that can arise with psychiatric medication management, working with a child psychiatrist who has training and experience with childhood OCD and/or anxiety disorders is critical. As many youth experience only a partial response to SRI medication, children and parents should plan to supplement ongoing medication management with CBT, especially to support continued improvements.

For patients with severe OCD symptoms, expert guidelines recommend the initial combined treatment of SRI medication and CBT (Bloch and Storch 2015; Geller and March 2012). This therapeutic approach should be continued for a minimum of 12 weeks to allow for an appropriate amount of time for both medication and therapeutic effects to emerge. For children that respond to this intervention, SRI medication management should be continued for a minimum of a year with CBT slowly discontinued. Patients that do not exhibit a significant improvement with this combined treatment may consider switching SRI medications and/or adding clomipramine to the existing SRI medication regiment (Bloch and Storch 2015).

What happens if my child does not respond to treatment?

There are multiple combinations and permutations for the treatment of OCD in children and adolescents, and it may require several different attempts to find the specific treatment combination to improve the patient's OCD symptoms.

For instance, as described above, some patients may have a minimal response to weekly CBT sessions. Several factors can play a role in CBT outcomes (e.g., therapeutic rapport, homework compliance, patient participation in sessions), and as such, patients and parents may consider pursuing CBT with another treatment provider to re-assess the benefit of CBT. However, if weekly CBT sessions are not enough to reduce OCD symptom severity, more intensive CBT options may prove useful. For example, intensive outpatient CBT, partial hospitalization programs, and residential treatment facilities are capable and experienced in providing empirically supported care in severe cases of childhood OCD. Similarly, patients may also not exhibit a treatment response to SRI medications for a variety of reasons (e.g., poor medication compliance, insufficient medication dose). Patients and parents should try an SRI medication for an adequate duration (12 weeks) at a therapeutic dose before considering switching to another SRI medication. If a patient does not exhibit a treatment response to three or more adequate trials of an SRI medication, the addition of clomipramine to supplement the existing SRI medication may prove beneficial (Bloch and Storch 2015).

PART 2

Treatment for Childhood Obsessive Compulsive Disorder

6

COGNITIVE BEHAVIORAL THERAPY FOR CHILDHOOD OBSESSIVE COMPULSIVE DISORDER

Adam M. Reid, Joseph P.H. McNamara, Gary R. Geffken

Introduction

Obsessive Compulsive Disorder (OCD) is characterized by intrusive thoughts, images, and impulses that cause considerable anxiety and lead individuals to develop ritualistic behaviors that provide short-term relief from this anxiety. Cognitive behavioral therapy (CBT) with exposure and response prevention (ERP) is the established psychotherapeutic treatment of choice for youth (and adults) with OCD. The crux of this treatment is exposure-based techniques, where the patient is challenged to systematically face feared stimuli or environments as a behavioral experiment to see if the patient's feared outcomes occur as commonly as believed. However, other techniques such as challenging anxious thoughts, learning about the nature of OCD, and teaching the family how to support the child with OCD are also used. To date, more than ten large research trials have all shown the superiority of CBT over other psychosocial treatments and medications for youth with OCD. Specifically, these studies show that the majority of youth with OCD who receive CBT experience clinically meaningful reductions in obsessive compulsive symptoms after just 9 to 14 one-hour treatment sessions (McGuire *et al.* 2015).

The history of CBT goes back to the middle of the twentieth century when a new branch of psychology, called behaviorism, became a leading theoretical approach to understanding mental illness. This branch of psychology developed behavioral principles such as classical conditioning, which explained how an individual could learn to fear a harmless stimulus (e.g. a "contaminated" doorknob), and operant conditioning, which explained why a repetitive behavior such as hand washing could develop to reduce the anxiety that resulted from touching that doorknob. Despite this movement toward behaviorism, youth with OCD from the 1950s to 1970s were commonly treated with older, less effective types of psychotherapy and medications.

Dr. Victor Meyer, a psychiatrist who spent the majority of his career treating patients at the Middlesex Hospital located in London, first "broke the ice" in the early 1970s by proposing and successfully implementing early forms of what we now call CBT. Specifically, Dr. Meyer showed that people with OCD were helped significantly by systematically exposing them to things that they feared, while simultaneously preventing the person from doing her rituals. Clinical research over the last 40 years resulted in the highly effective treatment that we use today. The CBT approach to treating youth with OCD will be reviewed in this and the following chapter. The goal of these chapters is to educate parents, teachers, and other healthcare professionals about this effective treatment approach for youth with OCD. Recommendations provided are based on recent clinical research and the combined 40 years of clinical experience the authors of this chapter have in implementing CBT for youth with OCD.

Overview of CBT for OCD

Locating treatment

Despite its effectiveness, CBT is difficult to find. Commonly, traditional cognitive behavioral therapy is delivered emphasizing non-exposure techniques. Or, providers offer therapy that has not been established to work. Thus, it can be very challenging to locate a practitioner who provides CBT, especially in more rural areas of the United States. The shortage of clinicians who provide CBT can result in long wait-lists at specialty centers and force families to travel long distances to receive appropriate care. It is not uncommon for youth to present for CBT who have previously seen several other mental health providers who tried treatments other than CBT that were unsuccessful. Considering that OCD rarely remits without treatment and can persist for years if untreated, it is important for youth with OCD to access appropriate care as soon as possible.

A few strategies may help youth with OCD find CBT treatment. First, it can be helpful to refer to the website for the International OCD Foundation.[1] This website provides a listing of providers in each state that are likely to provide appropriate CBT. Additionally, it is important for youth and their families to advocate for CBT services in their

---

1   www.IOCDF.org

interactions with healthcare professionals. Jeff Bell (2007), spokesperson of the IOCDF and news broadcaster, wrote about his lifelong struggle with OCD in his novel titled *Rewind, Replay, Repeat: A Memoir of Obsessive–Compulsive Disorder*. He states that a major turning point in his life was when, after years of unsuccessful psychological and medication treatment, he started advocating to his healthcare providers that he desired CBT. This resulted in Mr. Bell being referred to a practitioner who provided CBT and helped him successfully defeat his OCD and return to his broadcasting career.

Although psychologists are generally more likely to have the most access to in-depth training in CBT during their schooling, effective CBT could be delivered by a psychiatrist, psychologist, nurse practitioner, clinical social worker, master's level counselor, and so on. The type of treatment being provided is more important than the type of provider. If treatment is not conducted in a similar manner to what is described in these chapters, then alternative care may be needed. Some practitioners have strong beliefs against doing exposures and deliver approaches to treatment that are not supported by research. For example, many providers may convey that exposures will make symptoms worse, despite a lack of research supporting this claim. In some cases, however, CBT may not be indicated. If a patient presents with OCD and another co-occurring disorder, it may be helpful to treat the other condition if it is more problematic or would interfere with CBT. For example, youth with problems with disruptive and oppositional behavior problems may have trouble engaging in CBT for OCD. Therefore, treating these youth for their problems with disruptive and oppositional behavior before CBT for OCD may be most helpful.

Treatment frequency

Treatment can vary in length based on the severity of OCD and other factors that could impact success. However, standard CBT generally lasts for 12 to 15 sessions, with sessions lasting about 60 minutes. These sessions generally occur once a week, however, a few clinics offer semi-intensive or intensive CBT where sessions occur bi-weekly or daily, respectively. In general, intensive CBT for youth with OCD results in faster symptom improvement compared to weekly CBT, although weekly treatment may help more in the long term. For those with severe OCD, intensive treatment may need to be followed by weekly follow-up sessions to increase symptom reduction and reduce the risk of relapse.

Medication

Selective serotonin reuptake inhibitors (SSRIs) are the most effective medication treatment for youth with OCD. While less effective than CBT, SSRIs result in a meaningful reduction in obsessive compulsive symptoms for approximately 40 to 60 percent of children with OCD. If a youth does not respond to an SSRI such as sertraline, there are few tested medication approaches beyond switching to another SSRI.

On the one hand, combining CBT with SRI treatment has been shown to be more effective than SRI treatment alone. On the other hand (Ivarsson *et al.* 2015), combining SRI with CBT treatment does not seem to be more effective than CBT alone. Overall, adding SRI to CBT treatment may not have an added benefit, but the combination of CBT and SRI treatment does appear to work really well for youth with OCD. This research was conducted by expert CBT clinicians and, thus, the benefit to receiving CBT and SSRI treatment may depend on the provider's expertise in CBT. Combined treatment may be also be warranted if the patient has severe OCD that hinders them from engaging in CBT or the youth and their family are unable to attend frequent CBT sessions.

Assessment during CBT treatment

The gold-standard measure of obsessive compulsive severity in youth is called the Children's Yale-Brown Obsessive-Compulsive Scale. This clinician-administered measure involves a symptom checklist that identifies which obsessive compulsive symptoms are occurring, as well as questions that estimate the child's overall symptom severity. The complete measure is often administered during the initial visit to a clinic or the first session of CBT to determine the severity of symptoms and intensity of treatment, while the symptom severity portion of the measure can be administered repeatedly throughout treatment to monitor treatment progress.

Treating co-occurring disorders

Youth with OCD and one or more co-occurring disorders generally benefit less from CBT than youth with OCD. For this reason, a thorough diagnostic assessment before CBT is required. This assessment can identify co-occurring diagnoses that may interfere with treatment outcome. While co-occurring anxiety disorders and tic disorders are generally not believed to hinder CBT for youth with OCD, disruptive behavioral disorders (e.g., oppositional defiant disorder), major depressive disorder, pervasive developmental disorders, and attention-defiant hyperactivity disorder have all been shown to interfere with symptom reduction during CBT. If one or more of these co-occurring disorders are present, CBT can still be highly effective if combined with other treatments geared towards those conditions such as parent training for oppositional behavior or behavioral activation or SSRIs for depression.

Course of treatment

The overall goal of the first session of CBT is to teach the youth and her family about OCD, including how these symptoms develop and how CBT can reduce symptom severity. Because of its importance, the remainder of this chapter will provide the critical information that should be covered during psychoeducation. Hierarchy formation, usually completed during the second session of treatment, involves brainstorming a list of various anxiety-provoking stimuli and creating possible exposures that involve facing these feared stimuli. As exposures are created, the patient rates how much anxiety, or subjective units of distress (SUDS), they believe the challenges would produce. These rankings are used to create a hierarchy of challenges that the therapist can use to guide treatment. Creating a hierarchy or list of increasingly anxiety-provoking situations is important to treatment success. Clinical research has shown children can more readily approach less anxiety-provoking situations in early treatment sessions. This builds confidence to approach more highly anxiety-provoking situations in later treatment sessions. After psychoeducation and hierarchy formation, the remainder of treatment follows a roughly similar template each session: homework review, introduce or review CBT principles, exposure design, exposure implementation, consolidation of what the patient learned from the exposure exercise, and homework assignment. The "nuts and bolts" of CBT, including hierarchy formation and exposure implementation, will be covered in detail in Chapter 7.

Psychoeducation during CBT

It is essential to introduce psychoeducation at the beginning of treatment. The purpose of psychoeducation is to help the patient and her family understand the mechanisms that lead to obsessive compulsive symptoms, as well as how CBT is effective at reducing OCD symptoms. Psychoeducation is required for successful treatment as it improves patient insight into their symptoms, reduces feelings of embarrassment and feeling different than other people, increases motivation for treatment, and provides a clear rationale for why this type of treatment is appropriate. It is hard to benefit from CBT if one does not understand what behaviors make symptoms worse, or if one feels ashamed to discuss certain symptoms because of not wanting others to know about it or doubting that CBT will help. Below, we will explain psychoeducation in a similar manner to how it would be explained during treatment.

What is OCD?

OCD is a neurological disorder that occurs in about 1–2 percent of children and adolescents. This means that in a school of 800 students, there will be approximately between 8 and 16 students who have OCD. OCD has two core features: feelings of anxiety and anxiety-reducing behaviors or thoughts. Feelings of anxiety result from "OCD thoughts" or obsessions, which are experienced frequently (i.e., often an hour or more a day) and are highly distracting, distressing, and often viewed as unreasonable or excessive by the youth (although not always). These thoughts can widely vary in content but generally are related to a feared outcome in the immediate ("these germs will make me vomit") or distant future ("thinking about the devil while reading the Bible will ruin my salvation"). However, the thoughts can also be related to what the youth believes is "just right" or a stimulus that provokes shame or disgust. Often, these obsessions are experienced as an image or impulse that is disturbing to the youth. These cognitions trigger anxiety-reducing behaviors, or compulsions, that are often repetitive in nature due the frequency that the thoughts are experienced. The behaviors generally result in lowering the risk of a feared outcome (e.g., washing hands reduces risk of getting ill), correcting towards what is "just right," or reducing the experience of shame or disgust. What can be overlooked by some clinicians is the notion that thoughts themselves can serve as compulsions. For youth with OCD almost any cognition, such as thinking of a special color or a certain image, can neutralize an obsession and reduce a youth's anxiety.

While the exact reasons youth develop obsessive compulsive symptoms is not completely understood, research has identified that there are both biological and environmental factors that predispose a youth to develop OCD. Due to a family history of psychiatric disorders or by genetic mutations, a youth may be more prone to develop OCD when exposed to life experiences that lead to the expression of these specific genes. Examples of these life experiences include a traumatic event, chronic stress (e.g., a child with a shy temperament who is constantly stressed by social interaction), or even infections. Sometimes youth with OCD will recall a specific moment that triggered their symptoms, however this is not always the case.

A youth with OCD will rarely have only one obsession or compulsion; rather a variety of obsessions and compulsions are experienced that may be very different thematically. Obsessive compulsive symptoms may be classified into general groups such as harm coming to oneself or others (e.g., fear of accidentally running over a stranger with a car and thus checking the mirrors for bodies while driving), undesirable sexual actions or urges towards others (e.g., fear of impregnating a family member and thus refusing to touch them), concern over breaking moral or religious dogma (e.g., fear that thinking about non-religious material during a prayer nullifies the prayer and thus the prayer must be repeated), a need for symmetry or having things "just right" (e.g., fear that having items that are not in a perfect row will cause discomfort that will not lessen and thus aligning the items), a fear or disgust in response to objects or environments that are viewed as contaminated (e.g., fear of accidentally consuming feces and thus repeatedly washing self and food to be consumed) and other miscellaneous symptoms that include superstitious beliefs and behaviors (e.g., believing that green is an unlucky color and thus only carrying coins rather than dollar bills). Avoidance is very common in OCD and serves the same purpose as a ritual in the sense that avoiding a feared stimuli or environment temporarily lowers anxiety. It is worth mentioning that obsessive compulsive symptoms often cross dimensions, such as someone who needs to do a ritual involving symmetry to prevent harm coming to a loved one.

After explaining these dimensions during psycho-education, the distinction between peripheral fears and core fears should be made. Often youth with OCD have one or two core fears that underlie most of the obsessive compulsive symptoms expressed. This could be a fear of being imperfect, living with uncertainties, a fear of losing a loved one, etc. The core fears of youth with OCD need to be identified so that treatment is not spent addressing only peripheral fears, leaving the patient at a high risk for relapse. Core fears can often be identified through a discussion with the therapist, but treatment should not spend time trying to identify why these core fears developed. Some approaches to therapy (e.g. psychodynamic) may focus on such understanding but this is not important in CBT.

Everyone experiences obsessive compulsive symptoms to a certain degree. Several studies have shown that obsessions and compulsions commonly exist in the general public. For example, a teacher in graduate school often provided the following story to exemplify this point. One day he was walking down a steep hill during a rainy summer day. A student who was riding his bike down this hill at a very fast speed flew by him, at which point he had the intrusive thought to stick his umbrella in the spokes of the bike to make the biker crash. The teacher had no actual intention to perform this act or any reason to desire to hurt the biker, yet this violent thought occurred. Individuals with OCD have this sort of experience throughout the day, except their intrusive thoughts cause extreme anxiety and can be re-experienced for weeks after they are triggered. It is important for the therapist to remind the patient that even the more embarrassing and socially unacceptable dimensions of obsessive compulsive symptoms, such as sexual intrusions, occur in the general public and have been experienced by many people sitting in the therapy office. For this reason, the patient can benefit by sharing any type of obsessive compulsive symptom because the therapist has "seen it all" and, in reality, the thought is just a thought and says nothing about the character of the individual (this type of reassurance is important to provide in early treatment but should not be repeatedly provided as it may become a compulsion, further reinforcing the patient's anxiety).

What caused the OCD and how will this treatment help?

The cognitive-behavioral model of "how" OCD develops is best explained by drawing the graph seen in Figure 6.1.

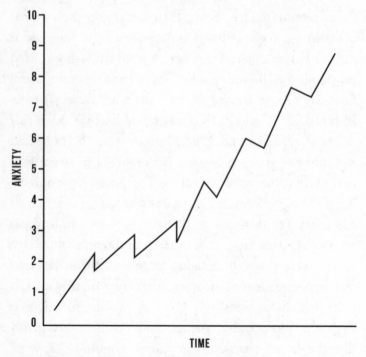

Figure 6.1 How OCD develops according to the cognitive-behavioral model

Anxiety is displayed on the y-axis and time is displayed on the x-axis. First, it is helpful to ask the patient what their favorite relaxing activity is and explain that a 0/10 anxiety is how she generally feels when she does that activity and is not worried about anything. On the other end of the spectrum, a 10/10 anxiety is how we would feel if a tiger was in the therapy room roaring and salivating from the mouth. This anxiety rating scale is identical to the SUDS ratings that will be used during exposure exercises to communicate to the therapist how anxious the youth with OCD is feeling. At this point, almost any obsessive compulsive symptom can be used to explain the remainder of the graph. Generally, it is easy to explain the model using a contamination example, although if the patient does not endorse any contamination fears then symptoms from other dimensions may be more useful. In the case example below, the graph is used to explain how contamination fears related to germs developed in a young adolescent who presented to our clinic with severe OCD and could pinpoint a time in high school biology class where her OCD was first triggered.

The first line in Figure 6.1 leading from 0 to 2 in anxiety represents the day in this biology class where she was using a microscope to look at the bacteria found on the school's bathroom doorknob. Viewing these bacteria caused a small but notable increase in her anxiety as she thought about how many times she had touched the doorknob. Feeling this anxiety and thinking about how she touched the slide that had these bacteria on it, she immediately washed her hands and decided to permanently avoid that bathroom at school. Immediately washing her hands and subsequent avoidance of that bathroom caused the anxiety to decrease, but not all the way back to where it was before this incident (indicated by the first downward-pointing line in Figure 6.1). Nevertheless, the drop in anxiety reinforced the hand washing and avoidance as effective short-term coping skills. However, avoidant thought (e.g., trying not to think of the bacteria she saw) and spending hours a day at that school (e.g., constant reminders of that bathroom doorknob) resulted in these thoughts repeatedly returning, resulting in more washing and further reinforced washing and avoidant behavior (represented by the second and third upside down check mark in Figure 6.1). Over time, since these behaviors appeared to have kept her from becoming ill, the thought of the bacteria caused even more anxiety and stronger urges to reduce this discomfort. These behaviors, while relieving in the short run, never fully reduce the anxiety to levels that they were originally before this cycle started.

Soon, the feared school bathroom doorknob generalized to any object in any bathroom, since these bacteria could be in any bathroom and were more likely to occur in places like the bathroom floor, flusher, toilet seat, and so on. The increase in the number of triggers resulted in a steep increase in the amount of anxiety experienced (represented by the steep line in the middle of Figure 6.1). As a result of the increase of triggers and the intensity of the obsessions, she began to wash more frequently and use stronger cleaning agents, such as bleach. It took her longer amounts of time engaging in these behaviors to feel any notable relief (i.e., the less steep lines going down in right half of the graph), but some short-term distress reduction is eventually achieved if more extreme efforts are utilized (e.g., wearing gloves in the bathroom). As this vicious cycle continued to worsen, she was soon convinced that her life was in jeopardy if she did not engage in an extensive ritualized bathroom routine (e.g., wear gloves that are bleached after use, wash hands for 20–30 minutes after each bathroom visit, only use personal bathroom at home). In essence, using the restroom had become as scary as facing that salivating tiger in the therapy room (i.e., the anxiety had reached a 10/10 on the graph). At the time she arrived for treatment, her fears had generalized enough to cause her to wear gloves throughout the entire day and multiple other contamination and non-contamination obsessive compulsive fears had developed.

To explain how CBT is effective in treating these obsessive compulsive symptoms, we find it helpful to draw another graph or add on to the graph shown in Figure 6.1. For the sake of clarity, we display this content in Figure 6.2, which is also shown in March and Mulle (1998). This graph shows how treatment intersects at the point where a patient typically engages in a compulsion in order to reduce their anxiety (i.e., where the prohibiting sign is displayed on the graph). At this point the therapist works with the patient to resist the urge to engage in a compulsion and rather sit with the anxiety until it habituates (e.g., reduces over time). Though anxiety initially increases during an exposure, habituation occurs both within session (i.e., indicated by the decreasing dotted line during each exposure) as well as between sessions when the same exposure is repeated (i.e., represented by the decreasing amount of anxiety elicited during repeated exposure trials). In other words, the patient will begin to feel less anxious during the exposure but will also feel less anxious next time she faces the feared stimuli. By fighting back against the OCD in this manner, the patient is able to learn 1) the feared outcome is not as likely to occur as previously believed, 2) she can tolerate the anxiety, and 3) the anxiety will reduce both in the short term (i.e., during the current exposure) as well as the long term (i.e., the next time she faces the feared stimuli or environment). The therapist uses various techniques to help the patient sit with the anxiety, expedite habituation and maximize learning, all of which will be covered in the next chapter. By engaging in this treatment process, the behaviors that became negatively reinforced during the acquisition process are no longer maintained by this reinforcement and decrease in frequency. The technical behavioral term for this decrease in frequency is called extinction.

After Figure 6.1 and 6.2 are reviewed with the youth it is important to remind her that she will be asked to recall these graphs throughout treatment. One younger child we worked with found it helpful to remember these figures by the phrase "lightning bolts and rainbows." It may be helpful to refer to these figures in this manner with younger children or any other way that will help the child remember what is to be recalled (e.g., take a picture with the patient's cell phone). After the rationale for CBT is presented, briefly mentioning the empirical support for CBT is helpful. This treatment approach has a wealth of support in the literature and is recommended by a variety of clinical organizations (e.g., American Academy of Child and Adolescent Psychiatry, National Institute for Health and Care Excellence) as the first-line psychotherapeutic treatment for youth with OCD. Providing this treatment rationale and reminding the patient of the research support is intended to increase treatment expectancy for the youth and her family, which would increase adherence and willingness to engage in the treatment process.

What will treatment be like?

Children and their families will often have questions about what it will be like for them to complete CBT. While treatment will involve completing exercises or exposures that cause an initial increase in anxiety, the exposures conducted will generally resemble experiences encountered on a day-to-day basis, especially during the beginning stages of treatment. The exposures will be conducted at the pace acceptable by the youth and she will never be physically forced to conduct an exposure. As the youth is asked to do more challenging exposures, she will have learned from easier challenges that will have prepared her for the more challenging exposures at the top of the hierarchy. An important point to make during psychoeducation is that the therapist will never ask a youth to do something the therapist would never do themselves. In fact, optimal CBT involves the therapist modeling whatever the exposure task is (e.g., eating off the floor), often doing more extreme versions of the challenge to model non-avoidance and maximize expectancy violations (e.g., the therapist who eats out of a garbage can should be ill at the next session).

At this point during psychoeducation, it can be helpful to conduct a "mini-exposure" to demonstrate the points covered during psychoeducation. This challenge should last between three and five minutes and should only elicit a very low amount of distress. Often the youth can brainstorm a challenge of this nature. This first challenge could involve the therapist and/or parent touching the door handle of the office door, rubbing soap on hands without rinsing, laying on the floor of the therapy office, etc. Before the challenge, a SUDS rating should be recorded. As SUDS are continued to be periodically recorded and anxiety reduction occurs (often just by one SUDS point since the challenge becomes easier), the therapist should highlight how this process occurred, pointing out that the youth now appears to be bored or having fun with the challenge. The treatment will follow this same process, where feared stimuli will become less distressing and even boring to the youth after exposure.

Psychoeducation for parents

While parents should be involved in all aspects of psychoeducation and ideally in treatment overall, some psychoeducation specifically for parents should be delivered during the early stages of CBT. The primary purpose of this psychoeducation is to address when parents unintentionally reinforce a child's OCD by helping her avoid a feared situation. This occurs when the parent engages in an activity that is in response to a youth's obsessive compulsive symptoms and the parent's behavior provides short-term relief from anxiety. The technical term for this is parental accommodation. Common examples of parental accommodation include providing reassurance (e.g., assuring that God will forgive a sin), enabling compulsive behavior (e.g., buying excessive amounts of detergent or hand soap), aiding in avoidant behavior (e.g., allowing the youth to miss school), or physically performing a compulsive behavior for the youth (e.g., rechecking locks). Parental accommodation is very common as parents may have a natural tendency to try to reduce discomfort their child is experiencing. When parents help their children avoid OCD related anxiety, they unintentionally contribute to their child's OCD, and may also decrease their own anxiety. From the beginning of treatment, parents should be encouraged to allow the youth to take the lead in her care (e.g., not forcing an exposure) but make it clear to the youth that they will systematically decrease the amount of accommodation they provide, at a rate that will be agreed upon during treatment.

Just as the therapist should be conducting all in-session exposures along with the patient, the parent involvement is equally important. Beyond modeling non-avoidance, this active involvement helps parents reduce their own anxiety that may contribute to accommodation. It also allows for the therapist to provide live coaching to the parent about how to respond to issues such as when the youth is resistant to treatment and how to respond to youth demands for accommodation. In this way, parents can also learn how to selectively provide attention for pro-treatment behavior (e.g., willingness to engage in challenges, homework adherence) and ignore treatment-interfering behavior (e.g., oppositional behavior, distracting behaviors).

Conclusion

In summary, CBT is the most evidenced-based approach to psychotherapy for youth with OCD. Psychoeducation is a critical aspect of CBT that occurs during the early sessions of CBT. Psychoeducation involves providing information related to what OCD is, how obsessions and compulsions normally occur in the general population, how OCD develops according to the cognitive-behavioral model, how CBT is effective in treating OCD based on this cognitive-behavioral model, and a brief exposure exercise to provide a live demonstration of the treatment principles reviewed during psychoeducation. Specific psychoeducation for the parents related to how to recognize parental accommodation and how parental accommodation can maintain obsessive compulsive symptoms should also be provided. Proper expectations should be conveyed during psychoeducation, including how effective CBT can be for the youth with OCD, what is expected of the youth and her family during treatment, and how the therapist and parents will be involved throughout the treatment process to provide coaching, emotional support, and modeling of exposure tasks. Appropriate teaching about OCD and its treatment lays the foundation for successful CBT. Thus psychoeducation is an element of treatment that cannot be skipped in an attempt to expedite the treatment process. Without psychoeducation, the reasons for engaging in the key aspects of CBT that are reviewed in the following chapter will be unclear to the patient and her family, increasing the risk for dropout or non-adherence.

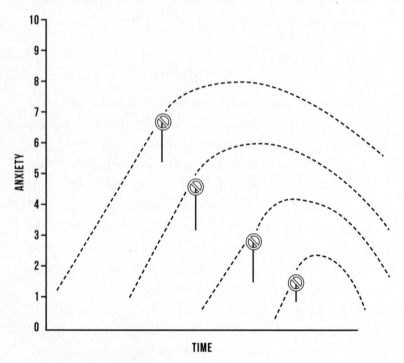

Figure 6.2 How CBT effectively treats obsessive compulsive symptoms

March and Mulle (1998)

7

EXPOSURE AND RESPONSE PREVENTION FOR CHILDHOOD OBSESSIVE COMPULSIVE DISORDER

THE NUTS AND BOLTS

Adam B. Lewin

Cognitive behavioral therapy (CBT) has become a "big tent" term for many talk therapies. Not all CBT is the same and the CBT approach for treating OCD differs from treatment of other anxiety disorders and depression. The key piece of CBT for OCD is exposure and response prevention (ERP) therapy. ERP should generally be mentioned (ideally emphasized) in the first sentence of describing psychological treatment for OCD. The key elements of ERP for OCD include:

1 psychological education (see Chapter 6)—rationale for the treatment approach and developing buy-in for the child and the family

2 fear hierarchy or fear ladder (developing a systematic approach for using ERP)

3 ERP—practice, practice, and more practice.

In addition to the ERP, CBT for OCD can also include cognitive tools for managing OCD (e.g., recognizing and challenging OCD thoughts), often depending on the child's developmental level. This chapter will cover some of the nuts and bolts of treatment—including hierarchy development and exposure and response prevention—specific to childhood OCD.

Building a fear hierarchy

What is a fear hierarchy (or ladder)?

The fear hierarchy (shortened to hierarchy from here on) is a ranking of OCD symptoms. For younger kids, describing the hierarchy as a ladder or staircase can facilitate understanding. See Figure 7.1 for an example of a fear hierarchy based on contamination fears; Figure 7.2 provides an example of multiple fear types placed on a single hierarchy. Obsessive compulsive symptoms perceived to be very difficult to change are placed on the top of the hierarchy and symptoms that the child is more willing to consider challenging with ERP are placed on the bottom. For example, a child with contamination fears may be willing to look at a picture of an overflowing trash can (low-level fear on the hierarchy) but the thought of touching the toilet bowl in a public shopping mall restroom would be extremely difficult (and placed on the top of the hierarchy). The hierarchy becomes a list for generating the easiest exposure and response prevention practices all the way up to the hardest exposure and response prevention practices, usually representing the easiest to most difficult rituals/compulsions to resist. It becomes the road map for ERP practice.

Estimated thermometer rating	Exposure task	Compulsion(s) to resist
10	Eating in the bathroom	Not swallowing cookie; spitting it out; drinking something right after; asking questions about cleanliness/ seeking reassurance
9.5	Touching the toilet seat	Inspecting the seat before touching; washing hands; inspecting hands; wiping off hands; avoiding touching things after
9	Scooping the cat litter	Holding breath; washing
8	Sitting in brother's chair	Cleaning chair; putting down a towel/placemat; asking parent to inspect it; avoiding eating
7	Shaking hands	Avoidance; poor contact; wiping off hand; using sanitizer; washing; avoiding food or touching phone/games
6.5	Using a drinking fountain	Spitting; inspecting mouth; rinsing; asking mom if it is "okay"
6	Opening doors at school with hand	Washing; avoiding eating; allowing others to open door— accommodation; using shirt or paper towel to hold handle; using elbow
4	Touching a doorknob at home	Washing hands; showering; avoiding touching things after; avoiding eating; asking questions
3	Using non-disposable utensils	Inspecting utensils; asking if it is clean; wiping or washing utensils
2	Petting dog	Washing; asking if it is "okay"
1.5	Wearing same socks to bed	Changing socks; inspecting socks; asking parent if it is "okay"

Figure 7.1 Example hierarchy/ladder—contamination fears

Estimated thermometer rating	Exposure task	Compulsion(s) to resist
10	Saying fearful "blasphemous" thoughts aloud	Praying; asking parents for reassurance; mental rituals
10	Eating foods that have been in contact with metal surfaces	Drinking water immediately after; inspecting food for metal shards; coughing to clear throat of potential "particles"
10	Holding a knife in the presence of parents	Asking "am I safe?"; avoidance behavior
8	Saying the word "vomit"	Doing mental ritual to undo fear
7	Completing homework without checking	Erasing; re-reading; seeking reassurance
6	Using a drinking fountain	Spitting; inspecting mouth; rinsing; asking mom if it is "okay"
5	Minimizing bedtime ritual	Telling parents that you love them more than once; continuing ritualistic entry procedure into the bed
5	Passing through doors	Continuing to pass through door an even number of times; continuing tapping door frame ritual
4	Alternate car seating	Sit on the "safe" side of the car
4	Wear school shirt in home	Changing out of "contaminated" schools clothes when returning home
3	Mixing foods	Not allowing foods to touch each other on plate; using multiple utensils at meals

Figure 7.2 Example hierarchy/ladder—mixed fears

Why make a hierarchy?

Just as one does not teach a teenager to drive on a busy Los Angeles freeway, teaching a child to manage anxiety works best starting with relatively easy ERP practices before moving on to the more difficult ones. Just as it is best to take the first driving lesson in an empty parking lot (on a Sunday morning), children find it easier to take on less scary obsessions and compulsions first. This promotes mastery and demonstrates that the tools can be effective—as well as seeming less scary. As the child adjusts to practicing ERP, it becomes easier to take on the more significant obsessions and compulsions that are further up the hierarchy. By conquering easier tasks and beginning to break the connection between obsessions and compulsions (see Chapter 6), those almost impossible tasks at the top of the hierarchy become less insurmountable by the time it comes time to challenge them. As the small dominos begin to fall, the big ones drop more easily.

How do you develop the hierarchy?

The hierarchy is a rank order of OCD symptoms. It is generally best to have the child start with the hardest (or easiest) OCD symptom he can imagine by thinking of a task that would trigger each obsession/fear, but then estimating how hard it would be to not do the compulsion for each obsession or trigger situation (e.g., touching a doorknob without compensatory hand washing). Visual-analog tools such as a "fear thermometer" can help to visualize this process—putting "high temperature" very fearful problems on top and "cooler," more manageable fears on the bottom (although most children these days have never seen an analog thermometer). For older children, Subjective Units of Distress Scale (SUDS) ratings can be done verbally, querying rating of fears as 0 (none) to 10 (extreme). The child and therapist can then work through a variety of symptoms to get as many tasks completed as possible.

It is best to generate a variety of situations that represent incremental gradations of OCD (e.g., with respect to time, frequency, or specific stimuli). It is important to produce low-level hierarchy items since these will be the first exposure and response prevention practices. If a child struggles to produce SUDS ratings, rank ordering is okay. Further, it is expected that adjustments to the hierarchy will be made over the course of ERP.

Exposure and response prevention

The goal of ERP is to break the connection between obsessions and compulsions, weaken anxiety, and strengthen the ability to habituate (or tolerate distress). ERP is based on the principle that the compulsions reduce the distress generated by obsessions, albeit temporarily. However, using compulsions (or rituals) to reduce anxiety actually "fuels" the obsessions and makes it more likely that the child will rely upon rituals as the go-to tool for reducing distress. During ERP, the aim is to trigger the obsession, but try to resist the compulsion. Over time and with practice, ERP should weaken the obsession (a process called extinction). The human body cannot stay anxious forever: without using a compulsion, the parasympathetic nervous system will eventually alleviate anxiety on its own (called habituation). Consequently, triggering the obsession and resisting the compulsion gives the child a chance to learn that the compulsion is not necessary and that the obsession will abate over time without ritualizing.

Figure 7.3 provides an example of this process. During the first ERP practice, anxiety rises and may take some time to decrease. The child then resists doing the compulsion and the anxiety eventually diminishes. Each time the same ERP practice is repeated, less anxiety/worry is generated and the anxiety goes away more rapidly. Thus, with repetition of a given ERP practice, exposure to the fear without using a ritual should result in both: (a) quicker habituation or calming and (b) lower initial distress (the situation should be less distressing overall). Notably, the first ERP practice may be difficult—the child may not experience significant reduction in anxiety. Emphasis should be placed on encouraging practice—not the reduction of anxiety. Just as the first time one picks up a violin there should not be the expectation that beautiful music is produced, the first ERP practice can be difficult and stressful.

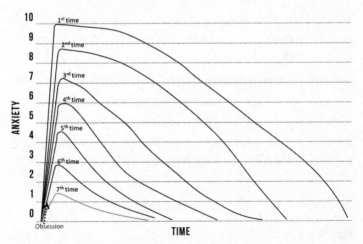

Figure 7.3 Exposure and response prevention

The first goal of ERP practice is to trigger the obsession (the worry or the scary thought) based on the hierarchy.

Exposures can be planned—and practiced incrementally. For example, in session, the child could be asked to put his hand in contact with increasingly fearful stimuli (and/or for longer durations, or more direct contact, or with longer delays before any washing). Especially early on, steps are repeated multiple times, demonstrating that the distress habituates more quickly with the practice. Alternatively, ERP practice can occur naturalistically. For example, certain "not-just-right" symptoms occur frequently with minimal need for creative planning. For example, a child that has to look at the left corner of a room after seeing the right corner of the room likely encounters the trigger in vivo without much need to recreate the experience. For these cases, it is best to plan out to which stimuli the child should target.

The second goal of ERP practice is ritual prevention: resisting compulsions in response to urges or distress. In some cases, the assignment is to resist the compulsion; in others it might be do the exact opposite of what it is perceived that OCD tells your child to do (e.g., touch the doorknob instead of avoiding it). Initially, this can be very difficult. The urge to complete the ritual is very strong, especially when the child has not yet learned that the distress/anxiety feelings will go away even without the compulsion.

Repetition

Exposure practice requires repetition: practice usually involves repeated exposure to the feared item (or situation) over and over again until the child's anxiety diminishes (and he can refrain from doing any rituals). Especially during early exposures, it is generally best to proceed slowly. It may be difficult for the child to resist at first—especially when the efficacy of ERP has not been demonstrated. Encouragement and praise for trying can be helpful at the early hierarchy steps. It is generally best to practice a particular exposure until the anxiety diminishes significantly more rapidly and/or does not elevate to the same extreme. Lower initial anxiety is another good benchmark for deciding when to progress. Therapists will base the decision to progress to the next step based on mastery, the child's SUDS or fear thermometer ratings, non-verbal behavior (complexion and posture can communicate a lot), compliance, and overall arousal. It is generally recommended to practice the ERP exercises done in a therapy session at home, even if it was mastered in the therapy session. Initially, progressing up the fear hierarchy is done in the therapy session, but eventually the child and family will learn to make decisions regarding how to undertake new ERP steps at home.

For some exposure and response prevention practice, it may help to take away anything that is needed to do a compulsion, for example, removing soap from the bathroom sink (for contamination OCD), or taking away the eraser on their pencil so that it is easier to not erase (for perfectionism OCD). For some youth, an early hierarchy item is to reduce reassurance (e.g., answering a child's repetitive questions that function as rituals). Many parents have trouble not answering their children and feel that by not answering they are making the anxiety worse. In actuality, providing reassurance maintains OCD—provision of reassurance is a ritual. In this case, the response prevention may be simply not responding to the OCD. Children are coached to recognize and reduce ritualistic questions and not respond to the OCD worries or thoughts. Parents should be encouraged to model "calm" behavior during ERP practice.

Especially in the cases of younger children, youth will look to parent facial expressions and other non-verbal behavior to judge safety. If parents look (or act) uncomfortable, it can make the experience more difficult for the child. Parents should be instructed to present a neutral expression during ERP—so as not to communicate surprise, fear, frustration, and so on.

Managing accommodation

Eliminating (or significantly reducing) accommodation of a child's rituals might be one of the primary ERP targets. In many cases, the parent becomes involved in ritualization, for example, by checking the child's hands to be sure they are clean or saying something "just right" or opening doors so the child does not have to touch the handle. Frequent, excessive reassurance is another example. More extreme examples may include taking your child to the emergency room to assure the child he is not ill or allowing him to avoid school. Sometimes, the participation is indirect: refilling soap every day, making special meals, extra loads of laundry, avoiding certain triggers. Removing caregiver and family participation in rituals can be part of the hierarchy. Accommodation is not discontinued abruptly. Instead, it's best to remove parental involvement in rituals gradually, using the hierarchy as a guide. Start with easier places to remove accommodation and work your way up. Some of this can be practiced during exposure practice. Other things are practiced when they happen in real life. For youth who resist exposure practice, gradually removing accommodation can be the best exposure.

Relaxation is not part of ERP

Unlike treating worries or fears that are not part of OCD, relaxation techniques are not recommended for OCD, especially while conducting ERP. Moreover, it is discouraged to have the child "try to think of something else" during the exposure (i.e., avoid using distraction). While it is natural for parents (and sometimes therapists) to struggle with seeing the child anxious or uncomfortable, the child should be encouraged to experience the distress and allow it to resolve without ritualizing. Parents should be coached to resist the temptation to help the child relax during the exposure. While initially it is permissible to encourage the child to resist the compulsion and to continue the exposure during ERP, it is best to minimize any conversation or attention during ERP. The therapist and the parent should avoid conversation in the child's presence during ERP as well. Following the exposure, praise is encouraged—even if the child remains anxious, his effort should be recognized.

Practicing in "real life"

It is important to use OCD triggers that occur throughout the day as an opportunity for frequent and "real life" ERP practice. Take, for example, the case of a child progressing through a hierarchy targeting contamination in which the child has practiced touching household items and not washing hands. The child has practiced touching toilet seats, brother's toys, the cat, mopheads, utility sinks, shower drains, etc. and now shows little anxiety and can resist washing. At that time, it becomes time to implement a rule: "hand washing only one time, when needed," for example, immediately preceding a meal or following a bowel movement. Specify rules and expectation (e.g., 30 seconds or less, one squirt of soap). If the child perceives the practice to be mild or moderate, the rule can be implemented. If the child expects extreme anxiety, it can be modified (e.g., allowing three "free" washes throughout the day or other modifications. Reassurance is another example. After being successful within session practice, an ERP assignment might be reducing (or removing) parental responses to reassurance. The child is tasked with not asking for reassurance and the parent is coached to ignore the requests. If necessary, reassurance can be phased out incrementally.

Using rewards

It is not uncommon for children to struggle with ERP so it can be helpful to use a reward program to help provide and maintain motivation. This is very helpful for younger children and similarly for older children who do not view OCD as a problem (or otherwise lack motivation). Reward programs can be implemented from the beginning of ERP, or started if the child is having trouble with participation. Rewards can be social (like words of encouragement, a hug, or a privilege) and tangible (like a new game or a special snack). It is generally best to make the reward only available for practicing ERP; it cannot be lost (or gained) for other behavior. Rewards may need to be changed if the child no longer enjoys the item or activity. Commencing with inexpensive or free rewards is recommended, for example: praise, hugs, special time or activities, getting to pick dinner. Engaging the child may be helpful in deciding the reward plan. The rewards are provided to increase participation in ERP—consequently, they should be provided as close to the participatory behavior as possible.

Cognitive techniques

Although ancillary to ERP, basic cognitive therapy techniques are often incorporated into CBT for OCD. For younger children, a helpful strategy is externalizing OCD as the problem, perhaps labeling OCD as a monster or bully. The child is coached to recognize the OCD and to "talk back" to his OCD. Self-talk aimed at bolstering efficacy, for example, "I know I can beat my OCD" or "I am stronger than my OCD" can be helpful. In other cases, simply labeling OCD "It's only my OCD," "My OCD plays tricks on me," or "I don't have to listen to OCD" can be supportive. For some youth, it can be helpful to talk about "fighting" OCD as a team, and discuss using ERP as the tools for battle. For youth more capable of abstraction, reframing worry as OCD can prove helpful. For example, "Nothing bad will happen if I don't do my ritual, it's just my OCD talking." Similarly, cognitive tools can be used as reminders, "If I give in to my OCD, it only gets stronger." For older youth, one can challenge OCD thinking, for instance, "How likely is [the feared consequence] to happen?" For example, "If you don't tap three times on the left then three times on the right after yawning, how likely is it that your mother will die?" Or another example: "Do you think I will die if I eat from an open package of breakfast cereal? I bet lots of people eat from open boxes of cereal every day without getting sick."

With OCD, it is important to be cautious when using cognitive techniques including self-talk. Some youth will replace rituals (especially reassurance) with self-talk (self-reassurance). In some cases, the self-talk or cognitive techniques can serve as rituals. It is important to remind the child that "anything that is making anxiety come down quickly might be a ritual." Consequently, it is important to tread carefully and ask youth about rituals they might be doing in their head.

Conclusion

OCD can be extremely disabling and burdensome for the entire family. Not surprisingly, when ERP treatment engages caregivers as well as children, the best outcomes are generally obtained. Cognitive behavioral therapy with ERP is the most preferred treatment by parents and has consistently proved efficacious for youth of all ages, even preschoolers with OCD symptoms. The fundamentals of ERP are relatively simple. However, it can be very difficult to engage and motivate children who are inherently uncomfortable with the idea of facing a terrifying fear without using the tools that bring safety or relief. Moreover, a number of children deny that OCD is a problem, lack insight into the irrationality of their symptoms, and/or present with a number of co-occurring problems such as depression, behavior problems, attention deficit hyperactivity disorder (ADHD), or Tourette Syndrome. In addition, family conflict and parental anxiety can complicate treatment. Nevertheless, children with OCD generally respond well to ERP, regardless of severity or other psychiatric problems.

8

TREATMENT-RESISTANT PEDIATRIC OBSESSIVE COMPULSIVE DISORDER

ASSESSMENT AND TREATMENT OPTIONS

Michael L. Sulkowski

First-line treatments

Once thought to be an extremely difficult-to-treat disorder, pediatric obsessive compulsive disorder (OCD) has been found to respond to very well to cognitive behavioral therapy (CBT) and to selective serotonin reuptake inhibitor (SSRI) treatment (Jordan *et al.* 2012). The Task Force on Promotion and Dissemination of Psychological Procedures (APA 1995) reports that CBT is a "well established" treatment for OCD—the highest possible rating—and meta-analytic research indicates that CBT has a strong effect (d = 1.45) on reducing OCD symptoms in children (Watson and Rees 2008). Similarly, compelling evidence exists for the efficacy of SSRIs to treat pediatric OCD. According to Geller and March (2012), every published placebo-controlled trial has found SSRI treatment to be superior to a pill placebo treatment.

Treatment-resistant OCD

However, despite displaying strong efficacy, some individuals still do not respond adequately to these treatments. These individuals are often called treatment resistant. They receive full and adequate trials of CBT and/or SSRI treatment, yet they do not experience a significant reduction in their OCD symptoms (Bloch and Storch 2015). Although they all share the problem of having a limited treatment response, some individuals display differences in the clinical issues and they present a challenge to even seasoned clinicians.

The International Treatment Refractory OCD Consortium (Pallanti et al. 2002) has proposed stages of response to treatment to determine treatment outcomes. A "full response" is defined as 35 percent or greater OCD symptom reduction on the Yale-Brown Obsessive-Compulsive Scale (Y-BOCS; Goodman et al. 1989), a well-established clinician-administered OCD measure, and a similar reduction in impairment on the Clinical Global Impression Scale (CGIS; Guy 1976), a commonly used measure of treatment response. In contrast, "partial response" is defined as a greater than 25 percent but less than 35 percent reduction of symptoms on the Y-BOCS and impairment on the GCIS. Lastly, "non-response" or a "non-responder" is defined as a person who experiences less than a 25 percent symptom reduction on the Y-BOCS and less than 25 percent in impairment on the CGIS. Overall, the Consortium defines "recovery" as a complete and objective disappearance of symptoms (i.e., Y-BOCS scores lower than nine) and "remission" as a response that reduces symptoms to a minimal level (i.e., Y-BOCS score of 16 or less).

Identifying treatment-resistant OCD

Research indicates that 46 percent of children who received combined CBT and SSRI treatment—an optimal treatment—did not experience symptoms remission in the Pediatric OCD Treatment Study (POTS 2004). Furthermore, many children who benefit from treatment still experience considerable distress associated with their residual OCD symptoms. Sometimes the improvements that many of these individuals experience do not hold across time.

Bloch and Storch (2015) recommend taking the following factors into consideration when determining cases of treatment-resistant OCD:

1 ensuring the right diagnosis

2 evidence of optimal delivery of CBT or medication, and

3 considering factors that can negatively impact treatment delivery and efficacy.

Several other psychiatric conditions display symptom overlap with OCD and have the potential to be falsely diagnosed as OCD (Geller and March 2012). For example, symmetry, ordering, and repetitive behaviors that often are observed in children with autism spectrum disorder can look similar to these behaviors in children with OCD yet serve different functions. Similarly, rumination associated with depression can also look like obsessive ruminations associated with OCD and delusions associated with severe mood and psychotic disorders also may seem obsessive.

Diagnostic accuracy

Ultimately, it is important to carefully diagnose OCD while ruling out other disorders that have symptoms that can look like OCD. Pence *et al.* (2010) discuss sub-optimal clinical outcomes in individuals who experience depressive episodes and psychotic symptoms during the course of treatment. Regarding the former, these individuals may feel unmotivated to continue treatment, or display an inconsistent treatment response during mood fluctuations. Regarding the latter, behavioral exposures can be misinterpreted as legitimate threats and cognitive restructuring likely will be ineffective with individuals who display delusional thinking and perceive the therapist as a person who has an ulterior motive (e.g., trying to exercise mind control, be part of a conspiracy plot).

Many diagnostic accuracy issues can be resolved through good communication between the clinician, child, parent, and any others who are involved in the child's care. Prior to initiating psychological or medical treatment, it is important for the clinician to be confident in the OCD diagnosis and to be able to rule out other possible diagnoses. Therefore, it is critically important for clinicians to receive information on the medical and psychiatric histories of children as well as for caregivers of children with OCD to be involved with assessment, treatment planning, and execution. In addition, clinicians should continually monitor the child's response while treatment ensues and carefully assess for untoward treatment effects. For example, if a child starts feeling so overwhelmed during treatment that she starts skipping or avoiding school, the therapist should focus on stabilizing the child to preserve her overall functioning (Pence *et al.* 2010).

Optimal delivery of a first-line treatment

Optimal delivery of a first-line treatment for OCD differs across types of first-line treatments. For CBT, this usually involves receiving an adequate dose of the treatment as determined by the number of sessions, length of the sessions, and what was actually done in therapy. In general, CBT should loosely follow a standardized treatment manual, occur during at least 45- to 90-minute sessions, be conducted on a weekly (or more frequent) basis, and last for a minimum of 12 sessions. Many practitioners report using CBT; however, variability exists with regard to what is actually done in treatment. For example, some clinicians may heavily implement cognitive restructuring (e.g., disputing cognitive distortions, challenging maladaptive thoughts) to the neglect of implementing exposure and response prevention (ERP). Although evidence exists for the efficacy of cognitive restructuring, component analysis treatment research indicates ERP has the most robust effect on reducing OCD symptoms (Chu *et al.* 2015). Therefore, it is important to determine whether an individual has received CBT with ERP and that the exposure tasks that the individual engaged in actually elicited anxiety. Experiencing and learning to habituate (i.e., become used to or accustomed to a stimulus or situation) to anxiety without having to perform anxiety-reducing compulsions is integral to the ERP process, a process that teaches individuals that they do not need to fear anxiety or obsessive thoughts or to engage in compulsions to reduce their distress temporarily (Jordan *et al.* 2012).

An established approach for treating OCD with SSRIs involves maximizing the tolerability of the medication (Bloch and Storch 2015). This involves starting individuals at a low dose of an SSRI and then waiting (usually between 8 and 12 weeks) to assess for a reduction in OCD symptoms. This approach is supported by findings that higher SSRI doses are associated with better outcomes for individuals with OCD as well as the relatively benign side effect profile associated with SSRI medication compared to other psychiatric medication options. Essentially, the goal of SSRI treatment for pediatric OCD is to maximize benefit and tolerability while slowly increasing the dose (as needed).

Bloch and Storch (2015) recommend against determining that an individual is resistant to treatment unless they have received CBT as well as two SSRIs at the maximum tolerated dose for an adequate duration of treatment (approximately 12 weeks) with the maximum dose being prescribed for at least eight weeks. In addition, it is important to consider whether an individual receiving combined psychological and medical treatments has responded to either treatment when considering whether they are a treatment non-responder. For example, an SSRI treatment-intolerant individual (i.e., a person who discontinues SSRI treatment because of side effects) might respond adequately to CBT and subsequently not be a treatment non-responder. Lastly, treatment compliance is an important consideration when determining treatment response. Whether assessing response to psychological or medical treatment, if treatment adherence is low (e.g., a child missed many medication doses, did not practice CBT), it is not possible to conclude that a first-line treatment has been received optimally.

Obviously, if a child did not respond appropriately to treatment because it was not implemented effectively, the first step is to try another treatment trial with proper integrity. Often generalist providers of psychology struggle to deliver first-line CBT treatment for OCD. Therefore, prior to classifying an individual as a "treatment non-responder," she should be encouraged to see therapists who specialize in evidence-based treatments for OCD.[1] However, these databases do not encompass all competent providers. Therefore, individuals seeking treatment can ask the following questions to know if CBT is being specifically tailored for OCD:

- Do you create an exposure hierarchy to help structure treatment?

- Does therapy involve homework and between-session practice opportunities?

- Do you discourage the performance of compulsions, avoidance, and escape behaviors during exposures?

- When necessary, does therapy involve "getting out of the office?"

- Do you involve important caregivers and partners during therapy?

If the answer to any of these questions is no, it may be worth seeking another provider who has more specialized experience treating OCD using CBT.

It is very important to work with an experienced child psychiatrist for medication treatment. Pediatricians or family medicine doctors, while well trained, often do not have much experience with pediatric OCD and may undermaximize medication treatment. These physicians

---

1 The International Obsessive-Compulsive Foundation and Anxiety Disorders Association provide databases of specialized providers who treat OCD.

receive generalist training in medicine so they can be effective at treating a wide range of conditions. Subsequently, as generalists, complex cases (e.g., children with multiple comorbidities, children with health and mental health problems) and treatment non-responders may be a challenge for these providers to manage. However, board-certified child and adolescent psychiatrists receive additional specialized training in child psychopharmacology. Thus, these physicians tend to be more familiar with treating pediatric OCD. They have to complete a multi-year postdoctoral fellowship in which they are supervised by a board-certified psychiatrist while they treat children and adolescents presenting with a range of psychiatric disorders. Thus, because of their additional training and competence working with child populations, it may benefit youth who do not respond to first-line SSRI treatment to see a board-certified child and adolescent psychiatrist.

Identifying factors that can impact treatment

Several factors have been identified that affect treatment delivery and efficacy for pediatric OCD. These include low insight into OCD symptoms, high family accommodation, and comorbid disruptive behavior disorders (Bloch and Storch 2015; Pallanti *et al.* 2002). Each of these variables will be discussed below as well as ways to potentially reduce their negative impact on treatment outcomes.

LOW INSIGHT INTO OCD SYMPTOMS

About one third of youth with OCD has low insight into their symptoms or fails to see them as irrational, excessive, or absurd (Lewin *et al.* 2010; Storch *et al.* 2014). Treatment for these individuals is then complicated, because they may not view their OCD symptoms as a problem. Instead, these symptoms may be viewed as necessary to feel safe or protect important people. For example, a child might develop a special prayer or mantra that she believes prevents something bad from happening to her or an important caregiver. When such beliefs are deeply entrenched then efforts to engage in treatment to challenge or reduce them likely will be frustrated. Essentially, ascribing to such beliefs can result in an onus to protect oneself or others from a perceived negative outcome as well as related distress.

Overlapping with low insight, Pence *et al.* (2010) reviewed cases in which CBT was used to treat individuals with OCD and low cognitive abilities. From this case review, the authors recommended modifying CBT for OCD for these individuals in the following ways:

1 increasing parental involvement in treatment

2 simplifying language

3 decreasing reliance on cognitive techniques, and

4 adding contingency management strategies and role modeling by caregivers.

Similarly, for individuals with low insight, CBT can be modified to be more concrete in delivery and important support people can be integrated heavily into the treatment process. Even if individuals have low insight into their OCD symptoms or do not see them as problematic, through the influence of key caregivers and by providing extra treatment-related incentives, these individuals may be willing to engage in CBT.

HIGH FAMILY ACCOMMODATION

Family accommodation of a child's OCD symptoms is associated with reduced treatment outcomes and greater overall family dysfunction (Bipeta *et al.* 2013). This phenomenon involves family members accommodating a child's OCD symptoms and participating in a dynamic that prevents the child with OCD from learning how to manage her own distress. For example, a child with contamination obsessions may demand her mother to wash her clothes immediately upon returning from public places and multiple times throughout the week. If the parent capitulates, the child will not learn that the feared outcome does not happen but also has reduced distress, making her try to get family members to accommodate further. Essentially, family accommodation is similar to a compulsive behavior that involves family members and subverts the habituation process that is integral to CBT.

Reducing family accommodation should be an important part of treatment for pediatric OCD and several studies underscore the importance of including caregivers in treatment (Barrett *et al.* 2005; Storch *et al.* 2007). It is important for therapists to identify this phenomenon and work with families to mitigate it. This can be accomplished through modeling exposure tasks in session with caregivers present; coaching caregivers to support the child with OCD—not the OCD; and helping caregivers anticipate, plan for, and effectively respond to an escalation in negative behavior (i.e., an "extinction burst") while they reduce their accommodation of OCD symptoms.

COMORBID DISRUPTIVE BEHAVIOR DISORDERS

The presence of comorbid disruptive behavior disorder (e.g., conduct disorder, oppositional defiant disorder) and OCD symptoms also reduces treatment outcomes. In one study investigating the impact of comorbidity on response to CBT for youth with pediatric OCD, comorbid disruptive behavior disorder symptoms were related to lower treatment response and remission rates (Storch *et al.* 2008). As part of their pathology, youth with comorbid disruptive behaviors are more likely to be defiant, potentially resistant to treatment, and to engage in problematic behaviors such as rage episodes that can interrupt treatment. In support of this notion, the severity of rage attacks displayed by youth with OCD has been found to influence impairment over and beyond OCD symptom severity (Storch *et al.* 2012). However, this relationship was mediated by the influence of family accommodation. Therefore, disruptive behavior such as rage episodes may contribute to accommodation of OCD symptoms, which may further increase OCD symptom severity and contribute to greater overall impairment.

Similar to modifying CBT to address the needs of children with comorbid tic and OCD symptoms, CBT also can be modified for youth with comorbid OCD and disruptive behavior disorder symptoms. To help children with the aforementioned clinical presentation, Rahman *et al.* (2013) recommend employing several different modifications to CBT for OCD. These strategies include treating anxiety/OCD symptoms as a primary indication, increasing motivation to engage in treatment, using contingency strategies to manage disruptive behavior while treating anxiety/OCD symptoms concurrently, and reducing disruptive behavior before initiating treatment. Thus, the overall focus should still be on mitigating OCD symptoms while also reducing disruptive behavior disorder symptoms as an impediment to treatment engagement.

Treating treatment-resistant OCD

People seeking treatment, caregivers, and therapists can feel frustrated and defeated when first-line treatments fail to work. However, several emerging and experimental psychological and medical treatment options still exist for treatment non-responders and treatment-resistant cases. In the remainder of the chapter, these options are discussed. More specifically, consistent with the focus of this chapter, both psychological and medical treatments for treatment-resistant cases are discussed. It is important to note that instead of being completely independent of first-line treatments, treatment strategies for treatment-resistant OCD often are described as treatment augmenters (Sulkowski *et al.* 2014). Essentially, these therapies aim to enhance a first-line treatment.

However, prior to discussing these treatment options, an important caveat must be acknowledged. This is that the majority of the approaches described below are still emerging and in need of additional research. Further, many of these treatments have not yet been rigorously tested and await further validation. However, as research continues to evolve, several of the discussed approaches may be reclassified from "experimental" to "established" or "well established." Thus, similar to how it took time to establish CBT and SSRI treatment as first-line treatments for pediatric OCD, it also will take time to establish effective treatments for treatment-resistant OCD.

Psychological approaches

Although CBT should almost always be a first-line treatment for pediatric OCD, research indicates that CBT can also be an effective augmenter for SSRI treatment for pediatric OCD. In the POTS II Study, a study investigating the augmentation of pharmacotherapy with CBT, the addition of CBT to ongoing SSRI treatment significantly improved treatment responses in youth with OCD (69 percent improvement relative; Franklin *et al.* 2011). In addition, youth who received CBT augmentation displayed superior treatment outcomes compared to youth who received CBT instruction and SSRI treatment as well as just SSRI treatment.

Similarly, a study by Storch *et al.* (2010) found compelling support for augmenting SSRI treatment with intensive CBT, which involved daily sessions for several weeks. More specifically, 80 percent of youth responded to intensive OCD and the majority of participants experienced significant symptom reduction at post-treatment. Intensive CBT involves seeing a therapist every day for three or four weeks. Thus, patients participating in intensive CBT receive a heavy and concentrated dose of therapy, which might have a particular benefit for treatment non-responders. Much of the benefit of weekly CBT for pediatric OCD is related to treatment compliance, which can attenuate with gaps between treatments. Because of the concentrated nature of intensive CBT, therapists can more quickly address treatment compliance issues as well as prevent backsliding between weekly sessions. In general, Bloch and Storch (2015) recommend using CBT as the optimal initial treatment augmenting approach because of its relative efficacy, high tolerability, and limited side effect profile.

CBT is considered a change-oriented form of psychotherapy. While engaging in treatment, people modify maladaptive cognitions and change problematic behavior patterns. Therefore, in order to have a favorable treatment outcome, people must be at least willing to entertain changing their thoughts and behaviors. Unfortunately, however, not all individuals with OCD enter therapy willing or ready to change, particularly if they have low insight, have a history of not responding to treatment, feel helpless to change, or feel like they are being dragged to therapy by a family member or partner (Maltby and Tolin 2005).

Instead of beginning CBT for pediatric OCD with patients experiencing the aforementioned problems, motivational techniques might need to be employed first. Motivational interviewing was developed to enhance motivation for change and resolve treatment ambivalence in patients with mental health and substance abuse problems (Miller, Rollnick, and Conforti 2002). Motivational interviewing has recently been applied to help individuals with OCD resolve ambivalence about change and engage in active treatments such as CBT. In one preliminary randomized trial, youth with OCD who received four sessions of motivational interviewing prior to beginning CBT displayed significantly better treatment outcomes compared to youth who received psychoeducation and CBT (Merlo *et al.* 2010). In addition, youth who received motivational interviewing completed treatment three sessions earlier on average when compared to the psychoeducation group, which provides preliminary support for the use of motivational interviewing as a treatment augmenter for pediatric OCD.

Medical approaches

Several different medical treatments have been used to either enhance first-line treatments for OCD or engage treatment non-responders. Some of these include using adjunctive D-cycloserine treatment, glutamate-modulating agents, and brain-derived neurotrophic factor; clomipramine (a previously established SRI treatment for OCD), yohimbine, atypical antipsychotic augmentation; ketamine, memantine, topiramate, and N-Acetylcysteine; and neurosurgical and neurostimulatory procedures (Bloch and Storch 2015; Sulkowski *et al.* 2014). Unfortunately, however, research on the efficacy and tolerability of these treatments with children is limited when compared to adults. In addition, many of these approaches are associated with serious and even dangerous side effects. Therefore, only the treatments with the greatest research base and current clinical utility will be reviewed in the remainder of this chapter.

ATYPICAL ANTIPSYCHOTIC AUGMENTATION OF SSRI TREATMENT

To date, research with adult populations generally supports the use of atypical antipsychotic augmentation of SSRI treatment for OCD (Bloch *et al.* 2006). In contrast, research in this treatment approach with children is currently lacking. In spite of this, augmenting SSRI treatment with an atypical antipsychotic medication may be worth considering for children who do not respond effectively to treatment because of positive findings in adult populations, particularly for cases in which comorbid tics and OCD symptoms exist. However, because of the side effect profile for these medications in children as well as the potential for poor tolerability, it is important to explore other more benign treatments first. Severe side effects are not common but include extrapyramidal symptoms such as pseudoparkinsonism (i.e., a reversible syndrome that includes tremulousness in the hands and arms, rigidity in the arms and shoulders, slowness of movement, loss or impairment of the power of voluntary movement, hyper-salivation) and tardive dyskinesia (i.e., an involuntary movement disorder that can occur with long-term antipsychotic treatment), as well as a lowered seizure threshold. More common yet less severe side effects include hypotension, sedation, weight gain, anticholinergic effects (e.g., constipation, urinary retention, dry mouth, blurred vision), and hyperprolactinemia (i.e., a condition of elevated serum prolactin). The prudent use of atypical antipsychotic augmentation of SSRI treatment is further supported by research suggesting that CBT outperformed this treatment approach in a recent randomized controlled study with adults (Simpson *et al.* 2013).

CLOMIPRAMINE AUGMENTATION OF SSRI TREATMENT

Research suggests that clomipramine, a tricyclic anti-depressant, is more effective at reducing OCD symptoms than SSRI treatment (see Geller *et al.* 2003 for review). However, clomipramine has a concerning side effect profile so SSRI medication is more commonly used to treat OCD. Some of these serious side effects include cardiac arrhythmia, increase risk of seizure, and fatal overdose in rare cases. Mild side effects of clomipramine include weight gain, dry mouth, drowsiness, and sedation. Despite being used off label, no randomly controlled trials have been conducted to evaluate the efficacy of clomipramine augmentation for

SSRI treatment in children with treatment resistant OCD. However, two randomized clinical trials have found success with this treatment approach in adults (Diniz *et al.* 2010; Pallanti *et al.* 1999). Therefore, more research clearly is needed on the efficacy of clomipramine augmentation of SSRI treatment for OCD, particularly in child populations.

USE OF TOPIRAMATE

Topiramate is an anticonvulsant or antiepileptic medication that is commonly used to treat epilepsy in children and adults. It also has been found to have mood-stabilizing properties (McElroy *et al.* 2014). In one randomized controlled trial conducted with adults, topiramate was found to be effective at reducing OCD symptoms in individuals who failed to respond to SSRI treatment (Mowla *et al.* 2010). More specifically, 50 percent of individuals receiving topiramate responded to treatment compared to 0 percent in a placebo group. However, these effects were not replicated in a second randomized controlled trial. Berlin *et al.* (2011) failed to detect a difference between individuals receiving topiramate and placebo in a sample of adults with treatment-resistant OCD. In addition, topiramate was poorly tolerated in this study as 28 percent of participants discontinued treatment because of side effects. Side effects for topiramate include fatigue, drowsiness, cognitive dulling, loss of coordination, and speech and language difficulties. Although the tolerability and safety of topiramate tends to be better than atypical antipsychotics and clomipramine, little is known about its efficacy for treating pediatric OCD. Therefore, caution is still warranted with the potential use of topiramate for treating children who do not respond adequately to first-line treatments.

USE OF GLUTAMATE-MODULATING AGENTS

Recent research indicates that glutamate abnormalities have been associated with the development of OCD symptoms (Kariuki-Nyuthe, Gomez-Mancilla, and Stein 2014). In light of this, increased attention has been focused on the potential for glutamate-modulating agents such as riluzole, a medication approved for treating amyotrophic lateral sclerosis (ALS; "Lou Gehrig's Disease"), to treat OCD symptoms. Findings in three uncontrolled clinical trials suggest that riluzole may be an effective treatment for OCD in adults and children (e.g., Coric *et al.* 2005; Grant *et al.* 2007; Pittenger *et al.* 2008). However, these findings were not replicated in a recent randomized controlled trail. Compared to a placebo control, riluzole failed to demonstrate any clinical benefit in a sample of children with OCD (Grant *et al.* 2014). Side effects associated with riluzole treatment include fatigue, dizziness, and nausea. However, in rare cases, riluzole also has been associated with hepatotoxicity (i.e., "chemical-driven liver damage") and pancreatic problems. Because of the conflicting findings regarding the efficacy of glutamate-modulating agents for treating OCD, Bloch and Storch (2015) state that these medications should only be used in cases in which other more evidence-based treatment options have been exhausted.

Neurosurgical and neurostimulatory procedures

Neurosurgical procedures for OCD are conducted only on the most treatment-resistant adult cases. These include the following ablative procedures: anterior cingulatomy, limbic leucotomy, capsulotomy, and subcaudate tractotomy. However, these procedures are rarely done with adults and should never be conducted with children. The OCD symptoms in children often remit over time, especially with the addition of first-line treatment(s). Furthermore, newer and less invasive procedures now exist that aim to accomplish some of the same goals as neurosurgery.

Deep brain stimulation involves surgically placing electrodes in key brain regions to deliver targeted electrical stimulation. This procedure is thought to regulate neurocognitive functioning, and it is reversible. Deep brain stimulation has been found to be generally safe; however, it is an expensive treatment and rare yet severe side effects can occur such as infection and intracranial bleeding. Even less invasive, repetitive transcranial magnetic stimulation is now being attempted with treatment-resistant OCD cases. This procedure involves applying a magnetic field to a patient's scalp to impact electrical energy under the underlying cortex. Unfortunately, despite having a favorable side effect profile, transcranial magnetic stimulation only reaches into the outer six centimeters of the cortex and it cannot impact deeper brain structures implicated in the pathogenesis of OCD. Research on the efficacy of the aforementioned procedures is emerging. However, to date, this information is limited with adults and almost non-existent with children.

Conclusion

Pediatric OCD, once thought to be an untreatable condition, responds extremely well to CBT and SSRI treatments. However, many youth do not respond adequately to first-line treatments for a multitude of reasons. Some of these reasons include problems with diagnostic accuracy, optimal delivery of a first-line treatment, and various moderators that can attenuate treatment delivery and efficacy.

When these problems are present, the first step is to adjust treatment to accommodate barriers to the success of a first-line treatment. However, when this is not possible or when individuals still fail to respond to treatment, alternative strategies may be attempted. Some of these include augmenting SSRI treatment with CBT, atypical antipsychotic medication, and clomipramine as well as the use of topiramate and glutamate-modulating agents. Lastly, in extreme cases, neurosurgical and neurostimulatory procedures have been attempted. As a final caveat, it is important to note that efficacy research is limited on the aforementioned treatment strategies, especially for pediatric cases. Therefore, considerable caution is warranted when exploring treatment options when first-line treatments have been exhausted for pediatric OCD.

9

FACTORS RELATED TO PROGNOSIS IN PEDIATRIC OBSESSIVE COMPULSIVE DISORDER

Jennifer M. Park

As noted in previous chapters, cognitive behavioral therapy (CBT) with exposure and response prevention (ERP) is the most empirically supported treatment for children and adolescents with obsessive compulsive disorder (OCD), followed by medication treatment with selective serotonin reuptake inhibitors (SSRIs). Despite the efficacy of these treatment options, a subset of youth with OCD does not respond to treatment. In general, variables such as gender and age do not impact how a child may respond to therapy or medication. Other variables, however, such as clinical presentation, family-related factors, and treatment-non-specific behaviors, have strong associations with treatment outcome, particularly in regards to CBT. This chapter will detail the various factors related to prognosis and discuss ways to maximize CBT with ERP treatment outcome.

Clinical characteristics

The clinical presentation of OCD can vary widely in regards to symptom severity, level of insight, treatment naïvety and multiple episodes, and co-occurring mental health conditions. Each of these areas should be carefully assessed prior to the start of treatment so that treatment may be tailored to account for each of these factors.

OCD severity

The severity of OCD symptoms before treatment is a reliable predictor of how well a child is likely to do. Specifically, those with less severe OCD prior to the start of treatment tend to have greater improvements following CBT with ERP (typically 10 to 14 sessions). The level of OCD severity can help guide which type of treatment and level of care may be most appropriate for the child. While professional guidelines for practitioners suggest CBT for mild to moderate OCD, a combination treatment of CBT and SSRIs is recommended for those with more severe OCD. Notably, recommendations are beginning to shift and increasingly CBT with ERP is being recommended first, even for many severe cases. This is consistent with a strong parent preference for behavioral treatments as well as evidence suggesting that even for youth who do not respond initially to CBT with ERP, extended courses of therapy may lead to similar results to that of adding medication to the treatment plan. The intensity of treatment provided for the child should also reflect the severity of symptoms. While weekly outpatient sessions are appropriate for mild to moderate OCD, more intensive CBT (i.e., longer sessions, greater frequency of sessions per week) may be indicated for severe OCD. Nevertheless, outcome studies suggest comparable results for intensive vs. weekly psychotherapy approaches. Thus, degree of disability (e.g., is a child able to attend school, maintain some social activities) and prior treatment response (success of weekly CBT in the past) should be considered when deciding the intensity of CBT needed. More detailed information regarding various treatment options and levels of care is discussed in a previous chapter.

Co-occurring psychiatric disorders

About 75 percent of youth with OCD also have co-occurring mental health conditions such as other anxiety disorders, depression, Tourette Syndrome and tic disorders, and attention deficit hyperactivity disorder (ADHD). Generally, having multiple psychiatric problems might predict a lesser response to treatment. However, research suggests mixed findings: depression and behavioral disorders seem to suggest that children may do less well with treatment, whereas having other anxiety may not have a negative effect on treatment. Findings are mixed regarding how tic disorders impact treatment. Clearly more information is needed to understand the impact of other psychiatric conditions on how well a child with OCD does in treatment.

In cases of co-occurring psychiatric problems, there is no one-size-fits-all approach regarding the order in which to treat symptoms. In some cases, co-occurring psychiatric conditions should be addressed prior to the start of treatment to maximize benefit. The presence of severe depression may increase feelings of hopelessness and fatigue, thereby decreasing motivation and energy to follow through with treatment plans (after all, ERP can require considerable energy, as youth are facing difficult fears while resisting strong urges). Initial therapy sessions can be focused on gradually increasing physical movement and activity on a daily basis and challenging negative and distorted thoughts related to depression to assuage depressive symptoms. While in some cases, managing depression first might be the best choice, at other times alleviating OCD using ERP (or an SSRI) can help lift a child from a depressive state. Consequently, many times the decision must be individualized to the child.

ADHD also presents challenges. Because distractibility and inability to concentrate is a core feature of ADHD, youth may have difficulty paying attention to and engaging with treatment; they may not absorb the skills taught in CBT or have the attention span to focus on exposure practices. During therapy sessions youth may need to be frequently redirected or prompted to stay on task. Additionally, those with ADHD may forget what their therapy homework is for the week, or they may lose worksheets that are given to them to complete for homework.

Oppositional defiant disorder is a condition in which children and adolescents are outright defiant towards parents and/or other adults by often refusing to listen to or comply with requests or demands, arguing frequently, becoming angry or annoyed easily, and/or throwing large-scale tantrums. Youth who are oppositional may not be willing to comply with treatment demands (e.g., practicing skills, taking medications on a regular basis). Behavioral management and parent training sessions, which focus on shaping behavior so that preferred behaviors (e.g., remaining calm or following through on tasks) are increased, are helpful for both ADHD and oppositional defiant disorder. Behavioral management sessions utilize rewards, such as positive attention from parents (e.g., praise), toys, games, and other activities to increase preferred behaviors, and use tactical or planned ignoring (i.e., purposefully ignoring specific behaviors) to decrease negative behaviors.

However, youth without oppositional defiant disorder may also show oppositional behaviors that are directly related to their OCD symptoms. For example, children may throw tantrums when parents refuse to accommodate or participate in their compulsions, or they may refuse to complete a chore because the activity will trigger their OCD symptoms (and they are unwilling or unable to tell parents that this is the case). In cases where oppositional behaviors are driven by the OCD, the treatment would first target managing the OCD symptoms and the family accommodation, rather than the oppositional behavior itself.

Insight

Insight is characterized by the individual's awareness that their thoughts and behaviors are due to OCD, and acknowledgment that these thoughts and behaviors are problematic to and interfering with their daily lives. For example, a child with hand-washing compulsions and good insight may readily note, "something inside of me tells me I'm dirty, even though I know I'm not and I feel like I have to wash my hands. I know it doesn't make any sense at all." Youth with good insight often find their symptoms troubling and are motivated to change. Good insight and motivation are positive signs as they indicate that the child may be willing to do what he needs for positive changes to occur (e.g., actively participate in treatment).

On the other hand, children and adolescents with poor insight will deny that OCD symptoms cause problems in their lives, or that the OCD symptoms even exist. A child with poor insight may state, "I don't see what the problem is. I wash my hands because they are dirty and need to be cleaned." Those with poor insight not only tend to have worse OCD symptoms, but also, the OCD symptoms cause more problems in their daily lives. For example, they may have more difficulties concentrating in school (completing homework, taking tests), enjoying their interactions with their friends and social activities, and getting along with family members. When children and adolescents are unable to acknowledge OCD symptoms as problematic or irrational, they are often unwilling to participate in therapy and practice ERP. As these youths will not acknowledge that these behaviors are problematic, they often do not believe that therapy is necessary. Because of this, poor insight can lead to a child's unwillingness to engage in or even attend therapy sessions.

Increasing youth's insight into symptoms can be difficult, but may be achieved through an ongoing discussion with the child regarding the consequences of the OCD symptoms. For example, youth can be prompted to identify the ways in which OCD symptoms interfere with their daily activities. ("Is there anything that you want to do that you're not able to because of these behaviors?"; "How much extra time would you have each day if you didn't do these things?"; "How would it make you feel if you couldn't do these things?"). Encouraging the child to document each time a compulsion occurs can also increase insight into their OCD. For example, a child with reassurance-seeking compulsions may state, "I don't ask questions that much, just a few times per day"; however, after documenting in a journal each time the reassurance-seeking behavior occurs, the child may realize that the reassurance-seeking questions occur over 50 times per day and may eventually come to acknowledge that this behavior is excessive and irrational.

Treatment naïve patients and multiple episodes

While not adequately studied, anecdotal evidence suggests that youth who are treatment naïve (i.e., those who have never received treatment, therapy, or otherwise for their OCD) will be more likely to benefit from and show improvement when in treatment. There are multiple avenues for treatment options for those with OCD. Children may start treatment with CBT with ERP. If substantial improvements are not made after 14 sessions, then the family may choose to extend the CBT sessions to several more months and/or add an SSRI to the treatment plan to boost the current treatment. Another option for a course of treatment can be to start with SSRIs. As there is no one-size-fits-all medication for OCD, youth may need to work through several different SSRIs before finding one that is the most effective in managing their OCD. Indeed, if improvements are not seen with one SSRI, this does not mean that another SSRI may not beneficial; therefore, it may take some time before the right medication is found for the child. Once a beneficial SSRI is found, CBT with ERP can then be added on to maximize the benefits of treatment.

Clearly the best-case scenario would be when a child has a single OCD episode and this episode is quickly identified and appropriately treated. Unfortunately, little is known regarding what may differentiate a child who undergoes treatment and experiences a full recovery versus a child who relapses. In depression, the more episodes of depression that have occurred in the past, the more episodes of depression are likely to occur in the future; it remains unknown whether this is the case in youth with OCD. However, clinical experience indicates that for those with multiple episodes of OCD (where OCD symptoms improve following treatment, and then return later on), who have made improvements with CBT in the past will be successful again in treatment.

Family factors

Family accommodation

Family accommodation refers to when family members actively participate in or facilitate an individual's OCD compulsions. For example, parents of a child with contamination symptoms may do extra loads of laundry each week to clean contaminated clothing or provide reassurance that an item is clean when questioned by the child. Changing the family routine because of a child's OCD symptoms is also a form of accommodation; parents may account for extra time between activities so that the child has enough time to complete rituals. Accommodation occurs in virtually all families of a child with OCD. Oftentimes, parents engage in these behaviors to prevent emotional distress or behavioral outbursts from the child. While well intentioned, family accommodation not only impairs the child's ability to function in an adaptive and developmentally appropriate manner, but also inter-feres with treatment. Indeed, youth have worse OCD symptoms when the family provides more accommodation. Furthermore, while in treatment, as families decrease their accommodation behaviors, the child's OCD symptoms improve.

Parent training sessions can be incorporated into sessions so that parents can learn to limit family accommodation in a manner that is most helpful for treatment. For example, children may balk if parents remove all accommodation immediately at the start of treatment. Instead, parents can slowly decrease the amount of accommodation provided each day (e.g., provide reassurance only five times a day rather than 20+ times). Additionally, parents can act as therapy coaches at home, reminding the child that accommodating compulsions will "feed" the symptoms and cause the OCD to grow, along with providing encouragement and support during these exposures.

Treatment non-specific factors

Treatment non-specific factors refer to aspects of therapy that are shared across most types of therapies. In other words, these are not elements that are specific to OCD treatment; instead, these are factors that exist in any type of psychotherapy that one might receive.

Treatment expectancy and preference

A parent's or child's expectations of treatment (i.e., perceptions on whether the treatment will be beneficial in targeting symptoms) can have a strong impact on how well a child responds to treatment. Some research suggests that when families expect to do better in treatment, they actually do better (perhaps due to better follow-through with CBT "homework" exercises). In other words, because ERP often requires the child (and parents) to actively engage in exposures (practicing a lot outside of the therapy session and integrating the practice into day-to-day activities), those who do not view the treatment as likely to be beneficial may be less likely to participate in exposure practices. To enhance treatment expectancy, education regarding how and why ERP practices are necessary to reduce OCD symptoms should be provided to families at the start of treatment and continuously discussed throughout treatment. Additionally, early successes with ERP in treatment can engender more positive expectations regarding treatment. In other words, if a child practices an exposure and is able to successfully reduce their anxiety early on in treatment, they will realize that these practices actually can help manage their OCD symptoms and this realization may increase their willingness to continue with the ERP practices. Because of this, it is best to start by practicing ERP with OCD symptoms that are low on the fear hierarchy (i.e., exposures that cause low levels of anxiety) to ensure that children are successful in their ERP practices.

Treatment preference refers to the type of treatment that parents prefer for their child, such as therapy versus psychiatric medication. Many parents prefer that their children receive behavioral therapy over medication, suggesting that parents feel more positively about behavioral therapy than medication, especially as a first-line treatment option. Parental attitudes towards the various treatment options guides parents' treatment preferences, and subsequently impacts treatment expectancy. If parents have a positive attitude towards behavioral therapy and prefer to explore therapy fully before trying medication, it is more likely that parents will expect that their child will do better in treatment and, therefore, invest more time and energy into the therapy. Because of this, it is important to take into consideration parents' treatment preferences when making treatment recommendations.

Treatment compliance

Treatment compliance refers to when a youth is willing to comply with what is asked of them in therapy, such as regular therapy attendance, active participation during sessions, and "homework" completion. Youth who are more compliant with treatment are also more likely to have greater improvements in their OCD symptoms. As ERP is the "meat" of OCD treatment, it is important that a youth is willing to participate and practice exposures during treatment sessions. Additionally, as mentioned previously, ERP related "homework" is assigned between sessions so that practices learned in session can be solidified and generalized to the outside world (e.g., school, home). As level of compliance, particularly homework compliance, tends to remain steady throughout treatment, it is important to emphasize to families at the start of treatment that good compliance is necessary to maximize benefits from therapy.

Therapeutic alliance

Therapeutic alliance refers to the relationship between the therapist and the patient. As children are often referred to treatment by parents (and may present to treatment unwillingly and/or with poorer insight), it is important for the therapist and child to develop a strong therapeutic alliance. Building a strong and positive therapeutic alliance can make youth more inclined to attend sessions and open up to their therapist about the difficulties that they are experiencing. This is especially important in the treatment of OCD as ERP can be difficult and, at times, aversive. It can be very helpful when feelings of mutual trust are engendered between the therapist and the child so that the child considers the therapy session to be a safe place where exposure practices can occur. Indeed, therapists, parents, and children who have reported a strong therapeutic alliance between the child and therapist have also shown greater improvements in treatment. The following case example demonstrates how to address some of these factors in treatment.

Clinical presentation

Andrew was a 13-year-old boy with contamination-related obsessions and compulsions. He believed that his school was a cesspool of bacteria and disease and that those contaminated from school may become severely ill. Because of this he made efforts to prevent school-related contamination from entering his home or "infecting" his family members. At the end of each school day Andrew placed school-related items (books, backpack, pencils, etc.) in plastic bags. Immediately after he entered his home, he removed the clothes he wore to school and showered for between 30 minutes and one hour (with the length depending on how contaminated he was that day). The contaminated clothes were placed in a plastic bag, which were laundered that evening by his parents. Following the shower, Andrew wiped down every area in the home that he may have touched on his way to the shower (e.g., bathroom floor, foyer, door handles). If Andrew believed that a family member may have been contaminated (by brushing by his school clothes or accidentally touching a contaminated item), that family member needed to also change clothes and take a shower. Andrew started to wake early in the mornings and clean areas in the house that he may have missed while cleaning the night before. On school days he refused to leave the home until these areas were thoroughly de-contaminated. When Andrew was not able to engage in compulsions or avoidance behaviors, he became extremely distressed and oppositional (e.g., yelling, crying, refusing to respond to prompts or commands).

Because of his OCD symptoms, Andrew's parents considered alternative schooling options (e.g., homeschool, therapeutic school). Andrew struggled to attend school on a regular basis and was often late or absent. To minimize the time he spent in school, Andrew quit the school soccer team and stopped attending debate club meeting and events. He was unable to complete his homework as he was unwilling to touch school-related items when home. His social relationships deteriorated as Andrew refused to allow school friends to enter his home as he believed that they were contaminated as well. Andrew's insight into his symptoms was poor. He thought that his cleaning compulsions were protecting himself and his family from sickness. He believed that going to a new school (and avoiding all contact from people and things from his old school) was a perfect solution as changing schools would subsequently cause his OCD symptoms to disappear. Because of this, he did not feel that treatment was necessary and was resistant to attending therapy.

Based on the evaluation, insight, treatment compliance, treatment expectancy, and family accommodation were identified as important areas to target early on in treatment.

Targeting insight

Due to Andrew's poor insight and unwillingness to start treatment, the first session focused primarily on enhancing insight into his symptoms and increasing motivation to engage in treatment. Andrew insisted his concerns were rational and his compulsions were necessary to keep his family safe. The therapist asked Andrew to think about the following: "What do you want your life to look like in ten years? Do you want to be doing the same things in the future as you are doing now (i.e., cleaning, washing, avoiding)? Are these behaviors leading you towards building the life that you want *in the future*? Are they allowing you to do the things that you want to do *today*? What are the things that you would do now if you could?"

Andrew noted that in ten years he hoped to be graduated from college and working towards becoming a veterinarian. He acknowledged should his OCD behaviors continue in the same manner, he would not be able to complete high school, preventing him from even attending college; however, he adamantly noted that changing schools (leaving his currently contaminated high school) would be the "perfect solution" to this OCD problem. He observed that his OCD symptoms were interfering with his ability to do the things he really enjoyed, such as spending time with friends and playing sports. Andrew admitted feeling depressed and hopeless because of the way his obsessions and compulsions have taken over his life. However, he continued to express the belief that as soon as he moved to a new school all these problems would cease to exist. The therapist continued to question this belief, drawing from his past experiences: "Did your symptoms disappear during winter break? What about summer break? If the symptoms did not stop while you were on break, why would it be different if you went to another school?"

Andrew admitted that even when he was not in school, he continued to wash and clean excessively. When gently pushed by the therapist, Andrew conceded that given that symptoms persisted when he was not in school, it was possible that even if he moved schools the contamination issues may continue. The therapist summarized the points of discussion with Andrew:

1 OCD makes you unhappy.

2 OCD keeps you from spending time with your friends, playing sports that you love, doing well in school.

3 Continuing to do things the way they are now (i.e., engage in OCD compulsions) may not allow you to reach the goals that you have for yourself, such as graduating high school, going to college, becoming a veterinarian.

4 There is a possibility that OCD may persist, even if you change schools.

Andrew was asked to consider whether he would be willing to try something that may be helpful in making his life easier and reducing some of the discomfort that he currently experienced. While still not completely sold on the idea of therapy, Andrew agreed to be willing to learn more about CBT for OCD.

Work with Andrew's wavering insight continued throughout treatment. The therapist encouraged Andrew to continue to observe ways in which OCD may interfere with his life. Through family-focused sessions, Andrew also developed more awareness of the stress imposed on his family members because of his OCD symptoms and the burden that family members felt due their participation in his OCD rituals.

Targeting treatment expectancy and treatment compliance

As Andrew's poor insight also contributed to his general reluctance to engage in therapy, the therapist was aware that treatment expectancy and treatment compliance would need to be addressed early on in order for Andrew to "buy in" to the treatment. The therapist made efforts to spend extra time during the education component of therapy to thoroughly discuss how ERP works, how these practices would be applied to Andrew's OCD symptoms, and answer any questions that came up. During this discussion, Andrew became worried when ERP was described to him ("the therapy sounds too scary"; "if I don't do my compulsions, I will be anxious for hours and hours"). The therapist assuaged Andrew's concerns by emphasizing that therapy would be a collaborative effort between him, his parents, and his therapist. The therapist informed Andrew that he would be "driving the bus" of therapy and he would never be forced to do something that he did not want to do. However, the therapist also made sure that Andrew understood that there would be times when he would be encouraged and pushed to go beyond his comfort level. The therapist told Andrew that while ERP seems very scary, the practices would start by targeting less anxiety-provoking OCD behaviors. The therapist pointed out the items that were the lowest on his fear hierarchy and noted that practices would start with the behaviors that he rated low on his fear thermometer. Andrew rated touching his old yearbook and refraining from washing his hands as a three out of ten. The therapist asked if he would be willing to practice this in session by placing the palm of his right hand on top of the yearbook for five seconds and refrain from washing afterwards.

Andrew was initially reluctant, so the therapist modified the exposure and asked Andrew if he would be willing to place just two of his fingers on the yearbook. Andrew agreed and practiced this ERP. He reported feeling a slight increase in anxiety (he rated it as a four), but then noticed that after a few minutes his anxiety quickly dropped down to a one. Andrew expressed surprise that his anxiety went down so quickly. The therapist then asked Andrew if he would be willing to do the same practice again. Andrew agreed, and again he noted that he felt his anxiety increase and then fall down again. These practices continued slowly in session until gradually Andrew was able to place his entire right hand palm on the yearbook and refrain from washing. For homework the therapist asked Andrew if he felt comfortable continuing these same practices at home with his right hand, and then also practicing with his left hand in the exact same way he had done in session (first with two fingers, then gradually working up to his entire palm). Andrew agreed. The therapist then emphasized again the importance of doing these ERP practices between sessions and asked Andrew to practice for five minutes per day.

Andrew returned the next session and reported that the ERP practices had become "boring" and that he could easily touch his yearbook. He showed the therapist by pulling out his yearbook from a bag and flipping through the pages with ease. The therapist asked Andrew to describe how the practices went; Andrew noted that the more he touched the yearbook without washing, the easier it became. The therapist highlighted this as a good example of why practicing ERPs between therapy sessions is so important. Andrew and the therapist continued to work through his fear hierarchy, starting with the lowest level items.

Whenever Andrew would show reluctance to do an ERP because of his anxiety, the therapist would remind Andrew of the success he was able to achieve with his first ERP practices with the yearbook. Through these early practices, Andrew was able to gradually realize that ERP could potentially be an effective treatment in improving his OCD and that regular participation in therapy would be needed to see the best improvement.

Targeting family accommodation

Education regarding the role of family accommodation in reinforcing and maintaining OCD symptoms was briefly provided to Andrew's parents during the first session. Andrew's parents were encouraged to spend time between sessions thinking of ways in which they may participate or facilitate rituals, or allow avoidance behaviors to occur. At the following session Andrew's parents brought a list, which included the following:

1 laundering Andrew's clothes on a daily basis

2 showering and changing their own clothes when Andrew believed they were contaminated

3 avoiding touching contaminated areas within the home and touching uncontaminated areas when they were contaminated

4 modifying daily routines to accommodate Andrew's rituals (e.g., being consistently late for work because they could not bring Andrew to school until his morning compulsions were complete)

5 driving different routes to avoid passing by the school when Andrew had left the house for

non-school related purposes (for example, to reach the grocery store, the fastest route goes by the school. Andrew had his parents go the long route to avoid passing by the school due to contamination concerns)

6 providing reassurance to Andrew that specific areas, items, and people were not contaminated.

This list was shared with Andrew and he stated that he needed his parents to continue to engage in these behaviors so that he could ensure that he could keep them safe. The therapist discussed with Andrew the ways in which these behaviors were actually hurting him, rather than helping him. While Andrew continued to have concerns, he agreed to include the family accommodation behaviors on the fear hierarchy when reminded that these behaviors would be targeted gradually and within a pace that he set himself.

From the various family accommodation behaviors, "driving by the school" was the lowest rated item on the fear hierarchy with a fear thermometer rating of three out of ten. Along with the exposure homework that Andrew was assigned to practice on an individual basis, Andrew and his parents practiced purposeful driving exposures. Initially, an agreed-upon time was scheduled for each evening where Andrew and his parents drove by the school. Andrew and his parents continued to practice purposeful exposures on a daily basis. Eventually Andrew agreed to practice "unplanned" exposures where Andrew's parents drove by the school without giving Andrew any advance notice. As the driving exposures became easier for Andrew to tolerate, Andrew's parents started to limit the number of times they provided Andrew reassurance to five times per parent, per day. Andrew's parents were coached to respond to Andrew's reassurance questions by identifying (to Andrew) the behavior as reassurance seeking prior to answering the question.

Family sessions continued throughout treatment and accommodation behaviors were identified as active treatment targets. Andrew's parents became more aware of subtle avoidance behaviors (e.g., Andrew said he was not hungry and skipped dinner, but actually he did not want to go out to a restaurant for fear of seeing a student from school) and added these behaviors to the fear hierarchy. Andrew's parents created firm boundaries with him and made efforts to readily identify and target any new accommodating behaviors that arose.

Conclusion

There are many factors that are associated with prognosis in youth with OCD. To enhance treatment outcomes, it is imperative that these factors are thoroughly evaluated and targeted when developing a treatment plan. Ongoing assessment of these factors throughout the course of treatment is necessary to tailor the treatment to fit the needs of each child. Sufficient time should be spent addressing potentially treatment-interfering variables and behaviors so to maximize treatment response.

10

DECISION-MAKING

TREATMENT OPTIONS AND LEVELS OF CARE

Robert R. Selles and Adam B. Lewin

Whether you're the parent who has realized that your child has OCD symptoms in need of intervention or a clinician evaluating a patient with OCD in need of specialized care, the following chapter is intended to guide you regarding what (empirically supported) treatments exist and how you can use a series of factors to determine what may be the optimal treatment.

Treatment options

The various components of treatment, the methods through which they work, and their viability in treating OCD are covered extensively in previous chapters, so will not be discussed here in great detail; however most simply, cognitive behavioral therapy (CBT), particularly that which employs exposure and response prevention techniques, is highly successful, leading to large symptom improvements in a large portion of youth. Further, children who complete CBT have been shown to maintain their improvement well past treatment completion (Barrett *et al.* 2005; Lewin *et al.* 2005a). As a result, CBT is considered the first-line treatment for OCD (Freeman *et al.* 2014). Most commonly, CBT is provided in an individual format (i.e., one patient and one clinician), involves family members, and is provided on a weekly basis. Research studies investigating CBT have frequently used a 10- to 12-session treatment protocol; however, in practice, the number of sessions may be more targeted to the individual's symptom severity and progress. Many variations on CBT delivery have also been investigated, and generally exhibit comparable efficacy, although their research basis is less well developed than individual outpatient CBT (Freeman *et al.* 2014). Group outpatient CBT, which employs the same components as individual CBT but has patients meet within a group of children with OCD, has generally exhibited comparable treatment effects to individual care (Jaurrieta *et al.* 2008; Jonsson and Hougaard 2009). The frequency of outpatient CBT has also been modified, for example, into intensive three weeks of daily one-hour sessions, with children experiencing similar improvements to weekly CBT, particularly at follow-up (Lewin *et al.* 2005b). Treatment can also be delivered on a more intensive basis, for example, multiple-hour daily programs or at residential/inpatient care programs. While overall treatment time increases in these programs, there is no clear method for deciding the best intensity treatment at which a child should begin. In other words, studies do not demonstrate that "more CBT" or more intensive CBT produce better outcomes. In fact, response rates were high in a recent truncated ten-session treatment protocol for youth with OCD. Thus, it is generally recommended to start with once-weekly CBT with ERP unless access to care is difficult or the level of disability is extremely high (e.g., not eating, not able to attend school).

In order to provide access to therapy for patients who live in areas without qualified therapists, investigators have looked at online and telephone delivery of CBT and found positive initial results (Comer *et al.* 2014; Storch *et al.* 2011; Turner *et al.* 2014). Further reducing therapist involvement, self-help books (referred to as bibliotherapy) have been developed that can be used in conjunction with minimal therapist involvement and without any therapist involvement. Stepped care approaches, in which low-intensity treatments (e.g., bibliotherapy, a few therapy sessions) are attempted first, then "stepping up" care to higher intensity treatment (e.g., weekly therapy or intensive therapy) may help improve access to care and reduce cost and difficulty placed on families (e.g., frequent therapy visits). Regarding pharmacological treatments, antidepressant medications, namely selective serotonin reuptake inhibitors (SSRIs), also are efficacious (Lewin *et al.* 2005b; POTS 2004) but parents generally prefer behavioral treatments (Lewin *et al.* 2014).

Decision-making

Level of severity and impairment

In a therapy utopia, where all treatment options are equally available, affordable, and effective, decisions regarding the level of care a child receives would be based on the severity of, and impairment resulting from, the child's symptoms. In medication management, a psychiatrist attempts to determine the level of medication that provides the ideal balance between benefit and risk. This model also applies to psychosocial treatments, in that the goal is to achieve the appropriate intervention dosage, providing enough support to be effective without over expending resources or causing additional difficulties. To illustrate this, let's use a case example:

Caleb has moderate-severe OCD symptoms primarily focused on fears of contamination. He obsesses, avoids, and engages in compulsions for multiple hours a day and has an extensive list of triggers, including a general fear of dirt and germs and specific foods, people, and places. Caleb is typically a compliant child, but has "meltdowns" when demands are set that trigger obsessions or prevent compulsions. Regarding impairment, Caleb is still attending and performing relatively well in school and is still capable of completing many things required of him, but his symptoms are putting significant stress on the family, particularly with Caleb's grandmother who Caleb believes to be contaminated, and have led to withdrawal from baseball and minimal contact with peers. In need of help, Caleb's parents search online and find that self-help treatment manuals are available for purchase online. In addition, within 30 minutes of their home they locate an outpatient clinician specializing in treating OCD, as well as a specialty center that has an intensive outpatient programme (IOP).

Scenario 1: Caleb's parents decide that seeing a therapist isn't needed, so they purchase the parent-focused self-help manual. Using the manual as a guide, Caleb's parents try to guide Caleb through some exposure and response prevention tasks. They collaborate with Caleb and choose a task they all think will be easy: touching the sink counter without washing hands after. Unfortunately, Caleb quickly becomes overwhelmed and says he has to wash his hands.

While they attempt to reason with Caleb that he should try not to, his behavior escalates and he begins crying and screaming. Unable to handle the level of distress their son is experiencing and unsure of the long-term outcome of such an event, they give in and allow Caleb to wash his hands, reinforcing the behavior. Further, they become disillusioned with attempting to confront symptoms and continue accommodating Caleb's symptoms.

Scenario 2: Believing that Caleb's symptoms warrant professional intervention, Caleb's parents pursue treatment through the outpatient clinician. Over the first six weeks in therapy Caleb continues to struggle. However, after a few successful exposures in week seven Caleb begins to demonstrate a considerable response and is significantly improved after 12 weeks in therapy. During this time, his schoolwork is minimally disrupted, and his parents are able to maintain regular work schedules.

Scenario 3: Believing that his symptoms need to be resolved immediately and that an intensive treatment must be better, Caleb's parents enroll Caleb in the IOP program. In order to make it work, Caleb must leave school at lunch each day and his mother and father must alternate taking time off work in order to accompany him. Caleb does well in the program and his symptoms have significantly improved by the end of three weeks; however, the missed school time results is a significant back-log of work and a reduction in Caleb's school performance, while the time off work puts financial strain on the family.

While it is impossible to predict with certainty which treatment level is perfect for each child (some children may do well in any level), this case example illustrates how severity and impairment can be used to zone in on the seeming "best fit" by illustrating how both too low and too high a dose can be problematic. The illustration is not intended as a comment on the value of treatments and with small changes to the level of severity and impairment, a different recommendation may be appropriate. For example, by reducing the number of triggers and level of distress, and Caleb's parents may have been successful in guiding exposures and could have experienced significant benefit from a minimal and low-cost intervention. Conversely, increasing the school-related impairment (e.g., not completing work, missing school time, failing), and the disruptive nature of an intensive program could be balanced out by the value of more immediate improvements in symptoms.

Individuals, whether the child, parent, or clinician, frequently base their idea of how severe or problematic the symptoms are on the evidence and experience they have available to them. For example, the parent of a child whose symptoms have recently and suddenly onset may perceive them as being more interfering than the parent of child who has become used to and learned to accommodate their child's longstanding OCD. To provide a point of reference for the recommendations presented in this chapter, Table 10.1, which mirrors a common assessment tool used by clinicians who specialize in OCD, provides a guide to what symptom severity and levels of impairment generally occupy each descriptor.

Table 10.1 A general guide to symptom
severity levels and their descriptors

Severity level	Descriptors		
	Occurrence	Distress	Impairment
Mild or below	Occasional-frequent	Mild-moderate	Occasional or non-essential across multiple domains or moderate in one domain
Mild-moderate	Frequent but not highly time consuming	Mild-moderate	Tasks are more difficult or stressful, but overall performance is not significantly affected
Moderate	Takes up a meaningful portion of the day	Moderate-severe	Tasks more difficult, some accommodation may be required, and some tasks may not be completed adequately
Moderate-severe	Takes up large portion of the day	Severe	No longer manageable and has resulted in significant disruption in functioning (e.g., child is failing school, extensive family accommodation, and loss of peer relationships)
Severe	Takes up the majority of the day	Severe-extreme	Widespread, a large portion of tasks are not being completed (e.g., child has been withdrawn from school, significant family disruption, little social interaction), and significant parent involvement is required
Extreme	(Near) constant	Extreme	Impairment is so extensive that child is non-functional (i.e., not able to complete any required tasks including self-care, school, social interaction) and requires constant care

Even with this general guide to severity levels, the domains in which symptoms are impairing, or the ways in which others respond to symptoms, can lead one to conclude that a different treatment may be appropriate for children with the same overall severity. Let's take another look at some case examples with two scenarios in which children who have the same, equally severe, symptoms experience impairment in ways that may alter the ideal treatment level:

1. Sarah and Caroline are equally afraid of germs and won't use public bathrooms. As a result of her fear, Sarah is frequently taken home in the middle of activities and her family limits the places they go. Caroline does not share when she has to go to the bathroom and as a result can have embarrassing and problematic accidents. As a result, her family has completely stopped bringing her to activities and places outside the home and is considering withdrawing her from school.

2. David and Matthew both perceive their siblings to be significant sources of contamination. David's sister is very understanding and tries her best to keep her stuff out of David's way and does not bother him. They don't have a close relationship as a result, but still get along. Matthew's sister is more impatient with Matthew's demands and will occasionally trigger Matthew on purpose by touching his stuff or going in his room. As a result their relationship is significantly strained and putting a great deal of stress on the family as a whole.

While not drastically different, the scenarios demonstrate how children with similar symptoms may be in need of slightly different levels of intervention based on the way in which they are experiencing interference. For Caroline and Matthew, the need for immediate improvement may be greater and as a result, may suggest a more intensive approach to treatment may be warranted, especially if they are unwilling or unable to participate in weekly outpatient care.

Availability

Outside of the therapy utopia, availability represents the most common determinant of treatment options that an individual could receive. In general, the availability of therapy options, both in terms of their prevalence and their cost, tends to decrease as the level of care increases. It is likely that most individuals can locate and afford a self-help book from a brick-and-mortar or online retailer; however, for example, the most intense level of treatment, residential, is offered at very few facilities worldwide. For outpatient CBT, efforts to better train therapists in CBT are gaining momentum; however, in many areas, particularly smaller cities and rural communities, there may be few, or no, well-trained professionals. In addition, some trained clinicians may have limited payment methods (e.g., cash only) and as a result may be outside the affordable range for many families. While parents are likely able to locate some form of psychotherapist in their community, alternate forms of psychosocial treatment (e.g., talk therapy, play therapy, psychoanalysis) do not have empirical support and many untrained clinicians may claim to provide CBT but are not well trained in the exposure and response prevention model central to the treatment of OCD. As a result, obtaining psychotherapy from these clinicians is likely to result in little improvement and, in some cases, could involve the encouragement of problematic behaviors. While the goal of alternative delivery methods for CBT and lower involvement methods, like web-based CBT, is to improve dissemination, these techniques are still in the early stages of development and may not yet be widespread. Further, while managed in a research study, the ethical and legal considerations of remote practice, particularly across state lines, are still being debated. Medication options tend to be easily accessible, as essentially all youth will have access to a medical doctor of some kind, whether pediatrician, family doctor, or psychiatrist, and insurance companies are typically willing to help cover medication costs.

To discuss the impact of these factors, here is another case example:

Beth has the same symptoms as Caleb; however, she lives in a smaller and more isolated city. When Beth's parents do a web search, they find that there are a number of therapists in their area, including some who say they treat OCD, but none who are well trained or specialized in CBT. With further searching they locate a psychiatrist in town, find a specialized outpatient therapist three hours away, and an IOP six hours away. If they choose to pursue local outpatient therapy with an unskilled clinician, they may spend many weeks in therapy without seeing any benefit and may see Beth's symptoms worsen during that time. They may desire specialized outpatient treatment, but traveling a large distance for one-hour sessions on a weekly basis is not feasible for their family and committing to travelling and staying near the IOP program would put significant strain on the family. Therefore, for Beth, web-delivered CBT could be an ideal starting point, but if not available, starting with medication may be a reasonable first step.

Preference

Patient preference (both child's and parents') is an important consideration in deciding on the appropriate level of care. If a family does not feel that a treatment approach will benefit them and is contrary to their preferences, they will likely exhibit reduced compliance to, and engagement in, that treatment. This may include poor homework compliance, inconsistent medication usage, and continued parental accommodation, all of which can be associated with reduced treatment outcomes. However, if a patient's preference is ill-advised given the child's severity and impairment, clinicians should not shy away from a frank discussion about the pros and cons of various treatment options and the importance of matching treatment dosage. Ultimately, the patient must choose what they feel is best; however, clinicians have the responsibility to ensure that their decision is an informed one.

Patient characteristics

As mentioned above, patient attitudes and behaviors can have a strong influence on the outcome of treatment. Many clinical characteristics, such as patient age, comorbid conditions, extent of accommodation, symptom type, and treatment history can influence the likelihood that a patient responds to treatment. Thorough coverage of important clinical characteristics, their specific effect on outcomes, and direct modifications that can be made to therapy is beyond the scope of this chapter; however, we will discuss the general influence these major clinical characteristics may have on selecting the level of treatment appropriate for a child. To do this, let's look at a few case examples that have various differences in some of these factors:

1. Mark is seven years old and Peter is 16 years old. Both have contamination concerns similar to Caleb. Mark, like many young children, has minimal insight into his symptoms, is reliant on his parents for many things, has difficulty maintaining attention to therapy tasks, and will be unable to follow complicated talk about therapy processes. Given this, having Mark's parents present for a large portion of therapy will likely be helpful to ensure they can help him understand, help monitor his completion of homework, and guide him during exposures. Peter on the other hand, has good insight into his symptoms, can easily understand the concepts presented during therapy, and is good at monitoring his homework completion. While discussions with his parents may be helpful, Peter would likely benefit equally from an individual approach.

2. Madeline and Alicia both experience intrusive thoughts about offending God. However, Madeline constantly confesses and seeks reassurance from her mother, while Alicia keeps the obsessions to herself and frequently engages in ritualistic prayer. Addressing Madeline's mother's role in the symptoms and eliciting her participation in exposure tasks will be an important aspect in reducing compulsions, compared to Alicia whose mother can only provide a supportive role in helping her tackle her exposures. As a result, it may be more important for Madeline to seek family-based treatment than Alicia.

3. Jeffrey, like Caleb has contamination concerns. However, in addition he is experiencing severe depressive symptoms including frequent suicidal thoughts and has occasionally expressed an interest in no longer being alive. Managing and adequately addressing these concerns may not always

be possible in weekly outpatient care and therefore a more intensive approach may be warranted for Jeffrey.

4. Brooke, Greg, and Andrew all have moderate symptoms appropriate for outpatient care but have the option to choose individual or group treatment. Brooke has fairly general contamination concerns, which are common to pediatric OCD. She may do well in a group treatment approach where, unlike individual treatment, she can benefit from seeing others with her symptoms (normalizes their occurrence), seeing others successfully complete exposures, and general peer/social support. Greg also has contamination concerns; however, his are very specific and uncommon. In particular, he believes babies may contaminate him and make him younger. He may be better suited to individual treatment since the exposures conducted in the group setting may not be as tailored to his concerns and therefore may be of less benefit. Finally, Andrew has obsessions that he perceives as highly embarrassing. In particular, he experiences intrusive thoughts about having sex with his family members. While Andrew may eventually experience benefit from having to share these obsessions in a group session, he is likely to have difficulty disclosing these obsessions initially to a group, which could lead to poorly targeted exposures or an increased risk of dropping out. As a result, Andrew may be better suited for individual therapy.

5. Taylor, Cameron, Abigail, and Lucas all have received treatment in the past but are still currently in need of therapy. Taylor is on antidepressant medication and has seen some benefit but is still experiencing problematic symptoms. He would likely benefit from initiating CBT, which has been shown to provide additional benefit beyond medication. Cameron completed an extensive CBT program in the

past and did not experience any benefit and has never been prescribed any medication. At the time of prior treatment, Cameron had very limited insight into his symptoms and, as a result, the therapist had trouble accurately targeting core fears. Since then, Cameron's insight has improved and he is better able to express his core fears. As a result, reattempting CBT could produce a treatment response. In contrast, Abigail previously failed to respond to CBT and there were no direct reasons to explain the cause, or changes in her presentation since, that would suggest treatment would work better at this point. For Abigail, consideration of an alternative delivery method (e.g., group versus individual) or consideration of medication might be justified. Finally, Lucas previously completed CBT and did very well; however, in the two years since he terminated treatment, his symptoms have returned. For Lucas, repeating CBT will likely be associated with great benefit and emphasizing response prevention techniques may contribute to better maintenance of his treatment gains in the future.

Table 10.2 summarizes some of these characteristics and how you may want to take them into account in deciding on an appropriate level of treatment for a child.

Table 10.2 Selecting the appropriate level of treatment based on certain clinical characteristics

Patient characteristic	Effect of treatment decision
Increased comorbidity	Increases importance of in-person approach May reduce suitability of group setting If severe or problematic, may warrant more intensive treatment
Increased family accommodation	Increases importance of family inclusion in therapy process
Decreased age, insight, or cognitive capacity	Increases importance of family inclusion in therapy process Increases importance of in-person approach
Increased symptom specificity/ complexity	Increases importance of in-person approach May reduce suitability of group setting
Increased parent contribution to symptoms (i.e., parent is contributing to symptoms via their own OC concerns)	Increases importance of family inclusion in therapy process
Prior unsuccessful attempts with medication	May indicate CBT is warranted
Prior unsuccessful attempts with qualified CBT	May indicate medication is warranted May indicate specific modifications to CBT may be needed to improve likelihood of response (see Chapter 11)

Stepped care

The right treatment for a child at treatment initiation may not continue to be the right level of care further down the road. As a result, for some children, it may be appropriate for a "step up" or "step down" in treatment dosage. The "step up" model has been developed in an effort to minimize the time spent by therapists with patients who will respond successfully with a lower dose intervention. In most studied applications of this strategy, children with severity levels on the lower end of the spectrum attempt bibliotherapy while being generally monitored for improvement. If improvement is realized the child continues with this strategy; however, if it is not, she is "stepped up" to outpatient care. This is a model that continues to be under research development and may not be commonly in practice in non-research settings.

The "step down" model is generally employed for children on the higher end of the severity spectrum that initiate treatment in high intensity programs like partial hospitalization programmes (PHPs) or IOPs. In these cases, often patients have improved enough to no longer warrant the cost and invasion of the higher intensity program, but still demonstrate a number of symptoms that warrant continued intervention. As a result, they may be referred to continue their therapy program at a level lower than their initial treatment dose. At an outpatient level, "stepping down" may simply involve gradually increasing time between sessions before therapy is eventually completely terminated.

Conclusion

With the largest evidence base, support for use across the majority of the severity spectrum, and reasonable accessibility, outpatient CBT represents the appropriate initial treatment for a majority of children. In addition, with continued efforts to vary the way in which outpatient CBT can be delivered, CBT will likely continue to grow and be accessible to a greater portion of the population in the future. Where any format of CBT is not available, medication often represents the most reasonable first step treatment option for families. More intensive programs, such as IOPs, PHPs, and residential care should generally be reserved for patients who have not responded to one or more full courses of CBT or CBT combined with pharmacotherapy, or who have symptoms that are highly debilitating, or have significant accessibility difficulties (i.e., it is easier to stay for three weeks somewhere far away than drive for six hours once per week).

PART 3

Considering Obsessive Compulsive Disorder at School and at Home

11

OBSESSIVE COMPULSIVE DISORDER AT SCHOOL

AN OVERVIEW FOR EDUCATORS

Lisa Bateman

Introduction

Obsessive compulsive disorder (OCD) can often directly affect children's educational experiences and overall functioning in school settings. Educators can play an important role in identifying symptoms that interfere with functioning at school and work with students, families, educational support staff, and treatment providers to ensure that these symptoms do not interfere with students' access to equal educational opportunities. In fact, researchers have reported that "teacher attitudes are critical to the success of students with OCD" (Leininger *et al.* Heath 2010).

Identifying OCD at school

Educators often play an important role in first identifying the symptoms of OCD that occur in the school setting and should therefore be aware of commonly associated symptoms of this disorder. After symptoms of OCD are identified, educators can begin to collaborate with parents, administrators, and mental health professionals to develop a plan to ensure that the student's symptoms do not interfere with the student's educational opportunities.

The first step for educators in working with students with OCD is recognizing the presence of OCD symptoms in the school environment. It is important to take into account that OCD symptoms can differ across home and school settings and that students may attempt to mask symptoms of OCD at school. In some cases, a student may have an OCD diagnosis but may choose not to disclose this diagnosis with educators. In other cases, because students spend such a significant amount of time in the school setting, educators may actually be the first individuals to identify symptoms of OCD before a diagnosis has been made. Given these possibilities, it is important for educators to be aware of common symptoms of OCD.

Although obsessions and compulsions can assume a variety of forms, there are some common obsessions and compulsions that occur in school-age children with OCD of which educators should be aware. Youth with OCD often experience obsessions related to contamination (e.g., fear of germs, disease, dirt, etc.), perfectionism (e.g., fear of making a mistake, concern about evenness or exactness, etc.), harm (e.g., fear of accidentally harming self or others), losing control (e.g., fear of acting on an impulse to harm someone else), and religious obsessions (e.g., fear of offending God, excessive concern with morality, etc.). It is important to note that youth with OCD can experience obsessions in addition to those previously listed, as an obsession can be any intrusive, recurrent thought that is typically accompanied by an uncomfortable emotion (e.g., fear, doubt, disgust, or a "not right" feeling). Educators should be aware of commonly occurring obsessions in youth with OCD but should also recognize that obsessions can occur outside of the aforementioned categories. It is also important for educators to understand that although a student with OCD may recognize that his obsessions are unnecessary or irrational, they are not within the student's control, and the student cannot simply "stop worrying" about the obsessions.

Because obsessions are internal, mental processes, it may be easier for educators to identify compulsions associated with OCD rather than obsessions. Youth with OCD exhibit some common compulsions, including washing/cleaning (e.g., washing hands or body excessively, excessive grooming or toileting routines, etc.), checking (e.g., checking for mistakes, checking for safety, etc.), repeating (e.g., re-writing, repeated body movements, etc.), mental compulsions (e.g., counting, praying, etc.), and seeking reassurance (e.g., from teachers, peers, etc.). Educators should be aware that not all repetitive behaviors are compulsive rituals. Compulsive behaviors can be distinguished from other repetitive behaviors in that they are done in order to reduce the anxiety associated with obsessions and/or to escape the presence of obsessions, and they are behaviors that the student may not want to do but feels driven to do in order to reduce anxiety associated with obsessions. They are often time consuming and frustrating to the individual because of the impairment that they cause in other areas of life. Like obsessions, compulsions are often difficult for the student to control, and though he may want to stop engaging in compulsions, he may feel unable to do so.

Not all compulsions can be observed externally, because students may perform compulsions mentally or covertly.

There are many possible indicators of OCD at school of which educators should be aware. These include repeated trips to the bathroom and/or spending an excessive amount of time in the bathroom during each visit; very rough, red, or cracked skin resulting from excessive washing; avoidance of certain places in the school that may especially trigger symptoms (e.g., a student who experiences contamination fears around food may avoid the school cafeteria); taking an excessive amount of time to complete work and/or turning in work with multiple erasures or holes in the paper from erasing; avoiding turning in work and/or consistently turning in work late; avoiding a certain number or certain tasks that may be associated with an obsession; excessive fidgeting with clothing and/or items in or on the desk; repeating tasks or starting over from the beginning if interrupted or if a mistake has been made; and repeatedly asking the same questions.

Educational impact of OCD

Students with OCD can experience a wide variety of educational challenges. Although they often have average or above levels of intelligence, the presence of obsessions may interfere with the student's ability to focus in the classroom, follow directions, and retain the material being taught. Moreover, students may not be able to complete schoolwork in the allotted time because of ruminating on obsessive thoughts and/or the need to perform compulsions, such as repeatedly checking work or repeatedly erasing and re-writing. Because of the presence of anxious thoughts surrounding schoolwork, students with OCD may also compulsively avoid doing schoolwork, homework, or even attending school and thus fall behind their peers. Often, avoidance of school-related activities becomes more prevalent over time because, as the student falls farther behind, he becomes more overwhelmed about the increasing volume of work to complete, and the pattern of avoidance becomes increasingly reinforcing.

Symptoms of OCD may also manifest as inattention, noncompliance, or disruptive behavior in educational settings. For example, a student who is experiencing intrusive thoughts throughout the school day may appear to be daydreaming or fatigued, and thus students with OCD may be at risk for being misidentified as having attention deficit hyperactivity disorder (ADHD). In addition, students with OCD may feel a need to perform a compulsion that contradicts with school behavioral expectations (e.g., frequently asking to go to the bathroom to engage in hand-washing rituals, repeatedly touching items after being told not to do so, repeatedly standing up and sitting down to perform a compulsion when the expectation is to remain seated, acting resistant to things that cause anxiety, etc.), and this behavior may be misinterpreted as noncompliance or defiance. Students who attempt to hold in their OCD symptoms at school may also experience anxiety attacks related to being unable to carry out compulsions that are typically done to reduce anxiety (Storch and Merlo 2006). Educators should also be aware that OCD commonly co-occurs with other disorders, such as ADHD, Tourette Syndrome, and depression, and should be familiar with symptoms of these disorders as well.

In addition to negatively affecting academic performance and adherence to behavioral expectations, symptoms of OCD can also affect students' social relationships at school. Students who are unable to mask compulsions in the school setting may be labeled as "different" or "weird" by their peers, which can result in social isolation and, in some cases, peer bullying. Students who attempt to hide their compulsions at school may exhibit increased frustration or behavioral outbursts when compulsions are unknowingly interrupted, or they may be perceived as controlling or bossy because they are unable to be flexible and react appropriately to situational and environmental changes. Students with OCD may also withdraw from peer situations or extracurricular activities in order to hide the symptoms of their OCD. Many children with OCD report experiencing difficulty making friends, keeping friends, and participating in developmentally appropriate peer activities.

OCD may also result in frequent tardiness and absences from school because of the amount of time that it takes for the student to perform rituals at home or the increased anxiety about being in the school setting. In some cases, OCD may manifest as school refusal. For example, a student with contamination obsessions may refuse to attend school as a result of fear of encountering germs in the classroom. At the most significant level of impairment, youth with OCD symptoms that are severe enough to require treatment in an inpatient or intensive outpatient program may need to take a temporary leave of absence from school in order to receive necessary treatment.

Treatment of OCD

In addition to understanding how to identify OCD, it is important for educators to have an overall understanding of how OCD is treated in order to develop appropriate educational plans for students with OCD. The two primary treatments for OCD with the most empirical support include cognitive behavioral therapy (CBT) with exposure and response prevention (ERP) and medication treatments, such as selective serotonin reuptake inhibitors (SSRIs). CBT has been consistently demonstrated through randomized controlled studies to be the most effective treatment for OCD compared to other forms of therapy and medications. Please see Chapters 6 to 9 for a full description of treatment of OCD.

If students and their parents/guardians agree, educators should collaborate with mental health professionals who are providing CBT in order to better understand the student's treatment. In particular, educators should be aware of the goals that students are pursuing in treatment so that they can monitor a student's progress (e.g., completion of exposures at school without engaging in compulsions or avoidance behaviors) and share these observations with the student's parents/guardians and mental health providers. For example, a student with OCD may be given homework assignments by his therapist to complete exposures in the school setting, such as touching certain items throughout the classroom to address contamination phobias. Educators can collaborate with the student and his parents to determine the exposures that the student is currently working on and support him in practicing these exposures in the classroom setting on a consistent basis. In some cases, students will be prescribed medication for their OCD. Although students and their families may choose not to disclose to educators that the student is taking medication, educators can be important reporters about the effectiveness of the medication in the school environment, as well as the presence of possible side effects. Feedback regarding symptom change as well as side effects (e.g., fatigue, changes in attentiveness, irritability) can help the provider decide on optimal dosing.

Interventions and accommodations for students with OCD

In the United States, OCD is considered to be a disability under federal law, and students with OCD are eligible to receive educational supports provided by the government for students with disabilities. In particular, the Individuals with Disabilities Education Act (IDEA) of 2004 and Section 504 of the Rehabilitation Act of 1973 provide protections for students who have been diagnosed with OCD. Parents and school personnel should collaborate to identify the unique needs of a student with OCD to determine the law under which it is most appropriate to seek services. In the United States, students with OCD may be eligible to receive special education services under IDEA under the category of "Other Health Impaired (OHI)" or "Emotional Disturbance (ED)." Under IDEA, students have access to Individual Education Plans (IEPs) with a diagnosis of OCD that has directly affected academic success or behavior despite the provision of tiered evidence-based interventions to address academic and/or behavioral needs. The intent of providing interventions at tiered levels of support is to ensure that students are receiving educational supports matched to their individual needs in the least restrictive environment. Interventions are often provided prior to the development of an IEP, and IEPs are typically considered when interventions are found to be insufficient in assisting the student in catching up with his peers or when interventions have been successful but need to be maintained long term for the student to continue to experience success. IEPs include specific data related to how a disability affects a student's educational experience, individualized academic and behavioral goals, and a list of accommodation and interventions identified to help the student achieve these goals. IEPs are generally developed by a team that includes the student's teachers, school administrators, a school psychologist, the student's parent(s) or guardian(s), and, for older students, often the student himself. Interventions included on IEPs may address academic goals (e.g., small-group instruction in specific math skills during the school day to help the student master skills that were missed because of frequent absences or impaired concentration), behavioral goals (e.g., implementation of a behavioral reinforcement system in which the student receives positive reinforcement for meeting a behavioral goal, such as reducing the number of daily trips to the bathroom to wash his hands), or social/emotional goals (e.g., implementation of school-based individual therapy to address symptoms of OCD). The provision of school-based individual therapy varies significantly across schools. In most school settings, a school psychologist or school counselor is present at the school several days per week, and this school professional can play an important role in collaborating with students' parents and treatment providers to determine the most appropriate way to support the student in the academic environment. Students with OCD may benefit from meeting with a school psychologist or counselor for support and encouragement or to optimize implementation of hierarchy-based ERP into the school setting. School psychologists/counselors can also play an important role in helping educators understand how to best accommodate a student with OCD in the classroom setting. OCD is often an exhausting, embarrassing, and intrusive disorder, and although it can be treated effectively, the treatment process is often stressful and frustrating. Regardless of if they are receiving treatment outside of the school or not, students with OCD can benefit from understanding and support on the part of school personnel. Interventions should be directly tied to the student's unique goals and should be based on empirical support.

Students can also qualify for accommodations in school based on symptoms of OCD. Accommodations are supports and services that are intended to promote equal educational opportunities. Students with OCD may be eligible to receive accommodations if their symptoms of OCD cause impairment in at least one major life activity as determined by a school-based team (e.g., teacher(s), parent(s), school psychologist, school counselor, etc.). For example, a student who is unable to complete a timed activity because of OCD symptoms that affect his speed (e.g., erasing and re-writing, re-reading, counting, etc.) could benefit from an accommodation of extra time to complete timed assignments until OCD symptoms have been addressed through mental health interventions. Common accommodations for students with OCD include the following:

- additional time to complete assignments

- testing in a different environment (e.g., a quiet environment, an environment without other peers present, etc.)

- passes to use the restroom as frequently as needed (especially for schools that have rules related to when and how often students are allowed to use the restroom or requirements that students ask before going to the restroom)

- preferential seating (e.g., being seated in the front of the classroom to minimize distractions and stress)

- having a "safe" place to go (especially for times in which the student is experiencing acute heightened anxiety)

- shortened assignments

- increased allowances to take breaks

- providing separate classroom materials for the student to use or allowing the student to pick materials first (for students that experience obsessions related to contamination)

- providing the students with notes or an outline of notes that were covered in class (if the student was experiencing difficulty maintaining attention because of obsessions and compulsions)

- providing materials (e.g., handouts, class notes) that the student missed due to tardiness or absences

- allowing the student to use technology (e.g., tape recorder, computer) to record notes in class (e.g., if erasing and re-writing interferes with the student's ability to efficiently and effectively take notes in class).

It is important to note that accommodations should be specifically matched to the student's individual needs and should only be implemented when appropriate and necessary to ensure that the student has equal access to educational opportunities despite his disability.

Medical and mental health professionals who treat individuals with OCD may express concerns that providing accommodations for symptoms of OCD in an educational setting may be inconsistent with techniques used in treatment for OCD symptoms (i.e., CBT) to help individuals overcome obsessions and compulsions. It is therefore important to carefully consider the provision of accommodations for OCD at school. For example, if a student is working in therapy sessions on exposures of touching "contaminated" objects without going to the bathroom to wash hands in therapy sessions and has been given instructions to continue to practice these skills outside of therapy, accommodations that allow the student to go to the bathroom as frequently as possible during the school day could be inconsistent with this therapeutic goal. However, it is also important to recognize that until symptoms of OCD have been appropriately managed through therapy and/or medication, students with OCD are at increased risk of experiencing academic and behavioral challenges at school and may require temporary accommodations to be successful in school. Educators should ideally establish ongoing communication with a student's treatment providers prior to implementing accommodations in the classroom in order to ensure that accommodations do not contradict goals established in therapy and to develop a plan for gradually withdrawing accommodations as the student's symptoms improve.

In some cases, a student with OCD may be required to take a leave of absence from school in order to pursue more intensive treatment options. In this case, educators should collaborate with families and treatment providers to establish the provision of temporary homebound services to ensure that the student's educational needs continue to be met while absent from the traditional school setting. For example, school districts within the United States offer hospital/homebound services in which educational needs are met through the use of virtual classrooms and in-home or inpatient visits from teachers who have received specialized training in providing these services. In the event that such services are provided, it is particularly important to also develop a plan for assisting the student in transitioning back to a traditional school setting once treatment has been completed. Ideally, educators should be in regular communication with parents and treatment providers to ensure that this transition is as seamless as possible. Some students may benefit from a gradual re-integration approach in which they return to school for some classes while completing some classes through virtual instruction options. All students would benefit from consideration of the usefulness of implementing temporary accommodations during this transition period. Educators, parents, and mental health providers should also address social issues with students as they return to school (e.g., how to respond when peers ask why they have been absent).

Conclusion

OCD affects at least 1 percent of school-age children and is associated with academic, behavioral, and social impairments that can affect a student's overall educational experience. Educators are uniquely positioned to identify symptoms of OCD and should be aware of commonly occurring symptoms associated with OCD. Once OCD has been identified, educators should establish ongoing collaboration with parents and mental health professionals to develop an individualized plan to ensure the student's success. Interventions and accommodations should be based on empirical support and should be tailored to the student's individual needs.

Tips for ensuring school success for students with OCD

- Ongoing, effective communication between home and school (and, if applicable and accessible, mental health treatment providers) is critical to ensuring student success.

- Educators may be uniquely positioned to first recognize symptoms of OCD because of the amount of time that students spend in schools, as well as the fact that some symptoms of OCD that do not appear in the home environment may manifest in the school environment. Educators should be familiar with commonly occurring symptoms of OCD and should establish clear communication with parents when such symptoms are observed.

- Symptoms of OCD may vary in different environments or at different times. They also may be misinterpreted (e.g., as ADHD, noncompliance, procrastination, defiance, etc.). It is important to understand the underlying cause and function of a student's behavior in order to develop appropriate and effective interventions. It is also important that teachers understand that symptoms related to OCD are not choices, and teachers should be careful not to ask students to control or resist behaviors related to OCD, as this could further exacerbate a student's anxiety about having to hide OCD symptoms at school.

- Accommodations may be necessary to ensure that a student with OCD has equal access to educational opportunities, but accommodations should be designed in collaboration with parents and mental health professionals to ensure that they promote the student's school success without interfering with treatment goals. If students are receiving treatment, accommodations should be gradually and appropriately removed as the student's symptoms of OCD decrease.

- Students with OCD may be at increased risk for peer victimization because of the obsessions and compulsive behaviors.

12

MANAGING OBSESSIVE COMPULSIVE DISORDER AT HOME

Brittany M. Rudy

Obsessive compulsive disorder (OCD) is a debilitating disorder that can have dramatic effects not only on the lives of those with the disorder, but also those around them. Families of children with OCD frequently experience interference in daily routines and family life. They also undergo their own distress and difficulty with handling and responding to obsessions and compulsions exhibited by the child. Unfortunately, OCD symptoms are often accompanied by disruptive behaviors and other, related concerns that impact parents, siblings, and family members and wreak havoc from day to day. Understanding and managing OCD and related behaviors at home is a challenging feat that is often overlooked in the treatment process. Factors such as accommodation of symptoms, reassurance, punishment, and treatment resistance can complicate the clinical profile of a child with OCD but are not always adequately addressed as part of the treatment plan. The purpose of this chapter is to provide parents and clinicians with information on ineffective and effective strategies for management of OCD symptoms at home as well as to discuss parents' roles in the treatment process, home practice, and maintenance of gains. This guide for parents and clinicians is written to highlight some of the ineffective strategies for and responses to OCD symptoms and to replace those strategies with more effective approaches for managing OCD at home.

Common ineffective strategies and their replacement approaches

Accommodation

A child's OCD symptoms typically affect not only the child, but the whole family as well. The rules, rigidity, fears, and routines frequently involve other family members and before long, the whole family participates in and works around the demands of the child's OCD. When this occurs, it is called *family accommodation*. Parents naturally feel anxious when their child appears to be in distress and will go to great lengths to minimize that distress. Accommodation occurs when family members change their own behavior in anticipation of potential anxiety or oppositional behaviors (or both) of a child. Unfortunately, helping the child to avoid anxiety or tantrums often increases the child's experience of OCD symptoms long term, and can greatly interfere with family functioning and daily life. For example, a child whose obsessions are on the topic of safety may have developed an elaborate bedtime routine that has grown and continues to grow over time. The routine may involve checking windows and doors, tucking in "just right," and having parents repeat special words before bed. This routine may seem harmless at first, but as the length grows (e.g., number of checks increases, number of words expands), and the inflexibility or rigidity with the routine increases, interference in family life likely also increases. As the parents allow the routine to continue in the same way and grow in length, participating in each part of the routine, the child's distress decreases and potential disruptive behaviors and sleeplessness are avoided. Unfortunately, the OCD symptoms are being accommodated and will continue to increase in severity over time extending the interfering nature of the routine. Similarly, if a child experiences obsessions surrounding germs and her parents wear gloves to prepare her food, re-wash plates, or allow extensive hand-washing rituals before each meal, these time-consuming and difficult processes may briefly reduce the child's anxiety and distress, but are complicating family routines, can prevent travel or dining out, and inevitably allow the OCD symptoms to gain ground. Such practices may seem beneficial or necessary when facing OCD symptoms, but can cause great struggles long term as the more a child uses avoidance or a ritual to relieve anxiety and/or ensure that things will go her way, the more likely the fear is to come back or worsen, and the more likely the child is to need to use the ritual, avoid the situation, or have things go her way to feel better again in the future.

Effective approach

Many families know that accommodating OCD symptoms is unhelpful at best if not frustrating, time consuming, and cumbersome, but reducing these behaviors is much easier said than done. When a child is not allowed to avoid feared situations or is asked to deviate from routines, her behavior may escalate (e.g., crying, tantrums, yelling, increased demands). In the short term, this effect can actually cause greater interference with family functioning than continuing the accommodation behaviors. For this reason, parents should work toward reducing accommodation of OCD symptoms in a gradual manner. Removing all accommodation at one time may be too difficult and distressing for the child and the family. However, reducing the timeframe or amount of avoidance, removing participation in rituals one step at a time, and enduring and appropriately disciplining (see below) disruptive behaviors associated with OCD symptoms, can be exceptionally beneficial for reducing the experience of OCD symptoms over time, as well as improving family life. Using the bedtime routine example from above, a parent would want to pick one aspect of the routine to reduce or choose not to participate in at first, then gradually continue to expand the reduction in participation. For instance, the parent may say that she will say the bedtime words once, but not three times (rather than not saying them at all). She may then set a time limit, stating that the routine (checking and all) must be done in 20 minutes. From there, the parent may consider encouraging the child to tuck herself in with less assistance. In this way, the parent does not completely deviate from the routine at once, but works gradually to reduce the time of the routine and the amount of participation. Similarly, the parent in the germ example from above may offer to fix a child's plate after washing her hands where the child can see, but not wear gloves. Before later meals the parent may offer to rinse the plate once but with no soap, and then not rinse the plate at all. Finding areas to reduce accommodation for less anxiety-provoking symptoms at a graduated pace can make a great impact on OCD symptomology and greatly improve quality of family life.

Excessive reassurance

Excessive reassurance or *over-reassurance* is a concept that is very similar to accommodation. Many children who experience OCD symptoms engage in reassurance-seeking behaviors and excessive questioning. For instance, a child who is fearful of germs may ask her mother if a yogurt is expired and/or is safe to eat prior to taking a bite. Again, this small act alone may seem harmless, but can grow in frequency and repetition very rapidly. When the mother responds by assuring the child that the yogurt is safe, the child's worry or distress is temporarily relieved, but the obsession over the safety of the food will quickly return. When this happens, the child will need to ask her mother more and more questions about the food and she may do so more than once, despite what the parent has already told her in previous responses (that the yogurt is safe). This is not due to a lack of trust or inattention, but rather because of the anxiety that the OCD symptoms cause. By excessively reassuring the child that the yogurt is safe, the mother is participating in a compulsive ritual, briefly alleviating the anxiety only for it to return. The conversation may look like this:

Child: Is my yogurt expired?

Mother: No, it is fine.

Child: Is it okay for me to eat it?

Mother: Yes of course.

Child: Are you sure that it is okay? Do you know that it is okay?

Mother: Yes!! I said it is fine!

Child: So it is okay then?

This type of conversation can also be very time consuming and over time can be tiring and frustrating for the parent. Generally, reassurance-seeking behaviors grow over time, causing parents to become a point of dependence rather than encouraging independence for the child.

Effective approach

Decreasing reassurance can also be a challenging feat. Some reassurance is necessary in a child's appropriate growth and development. Further, as parents, it is important to provide a safe base for a child and to be a place of comfort. However, as illustrated above, with regard to OCD symptoms, over-reassurance can be detrimental to OCD symptoms and cause greater distress for the child and parent over time. A good rule of thumb is to provide an answer to a question (especially one seeking assurance) one time only. Do not repeat the response. Instead, asking the child to find the answer or to reference the initial answer given is an acceptable response. Reverse questioning such as "Do you think your yogurt is okay to eat?" or "How could you find out?" is always a good technique. Additionally, it is alright to inform the child that a response has already been given and the question will not be answered again. Responses such as "I have already answered that question," or "I am only going to answer you once" can be helpful in informing the child of expectations and guidelines for asking questions and receiving answers. It is also a good idea to discuss with the child in advance of beginning the new question policy that future questions will only be answered once. Active ignoring—a strategy of fully ignoring the child while she is repeating questions and/or whining about receiving an answer—by turning away, avoiding eye contact, and even leaving the room if necessary, is a good technique to help reduce excessive questioning and accompanying reassurance. This process is likely to be difficult at first, but can help substantially with reducing OCD questioning rituals and improving critical thinking skills long term.

Punishment

Dealing with OCD symptoms in daily life can be frustrating for the child who experiences the symptoms as well as for the parents who often may struggle to understand the child's position or feelings, especially given the frequent illogical nature of the obsessions and compulsions. Rituals can be elaborate and time consuming and as mentioned already in this chapter, can interfere with daily family life. For example, if a child has developed an elaborate ritual over socks and shoes, this may cause difficulty with leaving the house on time each morning. Being late day after day may cause arguments between the parent(s) and the child over the socks and shoes, leading to frustration for everyone involved. Some parents may be inclined to provide punishment (e.g., removal of privileges, time out, spankings) for their children for ritual participation and resulting outcomes (e.g., being late to school). Although tempting, punishment generally is not a helpful strategy for reducing OCD symptoms and behaviors. It is important to remember that no matter how illogical or nonsensical an obsession or compulsion appears, the anxiety and distress associated with the obsession are real for the child, and the OCD behaviors are strong. Punishing a child may cause shame and further distress, as the child often feels that she cannot control her thoughts and actions, especially if the child (and family) has not participated in any treatment sessions and/or received education about the disorder. Punishment for the anxiety and rituals themselves may therefore increase stress within the family, without resulting in reduction of symptoms.

Effective approach: discipline— when is it appropriate?

While punishment of anxiety and compulsive behaviors is unhelpful, discipline is appropriate in certain situations related to OCD. Parents should understand that disruptive behaviors associated with OCD symptoms, such as tantrums, yelling, physical aggression, and refusals, are *never* appropriate actions and should always be met with an appropriate consequence. For instance, it is acceptable for a child who experiences a ritual surrounding socks and shoes to express distress at being hurried through the ritual or to be unable to put on her socks and shoes only once (prior to treatment and practice). It would not be okay for that child to refuse to put on the socks and shoes at all for school or to become angry and throw the socks and shoes at her parents. If either of those actions occurs, the child should receive an age-appropriate consequence for the refusal or aggressive action, but not for the ritual itself. Additionally, once treatment and home practice begins, refusals of participation in practice should be considered disruptive behaviors and disciplined as such; however, if a practice exercise is too difficult and the child appropriately communicates that, it would be important to find a compromise (see discussion of home practice below) for the activity rather than forcing the child into the overly difficult situation.

For younger children, the most appropriate form of discipline in response to disruptive or oppositional behaviors associated with OCD symptoms is likely time out. It is important to use a specific time-out procedure that the child understands in advance, through introduction in a family meeting, and to use the same procedure each time. Here is an example time-out procedure:

- Time-out chair:

  - Disruptive behaviors result in three minutes (plus five seconds of silence) in a time-out chair that is positioned in a "boring" area of the home away from walls and windows.

  - The five-seconds-of-silence rule implies that the child would be required to remain in the chair until quiet for at least five seconds. Therefore, following the end of the three-minute time out if the child is still making noise, the time out continues until the child is quiet and the parent can count to five in their head (not aloud). Inform the child that she could not leave the chair until quiet *before* the time out begins.

- Time-out room:

  - Should the child leave the chair prior to the three-minute duration, she would be required to sit in a time-out room for one minute (plus five seconds of silence) and then return to the time-out chair.

- A time-out room should be a small bathroom, laundry room, spare room with minimal distractions, or big closet area that is lighted and deemed safe for the child to be alone.

- Once returned to the chair, the three minutes (plus five seconds of silence) of time out would re-start.

- At the end of the time out, she would be required to complete the requested task or provide retribution (depending on the reason for the time out), before returning to play or other activities.

For older children, removal of privileges such as electronics or preferred activities may be a more age-appropriate option. One common way to set up such discipline is to provide an if/then statement as a warning to the child prior to or at the beginning of the disruptive behavior (e.g., "if you continue yelling, you will not get to use your iPad for the rest of the day" or "if you refuse to try the practice activity *specify activity,* you will not be able to go outside to play with your friends"). Parents may also choose to use punish work or chores for discipline, especially depending on the child's actions. For example, should a child throw an object and cause damage, the child may have to complete chores to earn money to fix the damage. Privilege loss is more common and more immediate, though natural and logical consequences (such as punish work) can be very effective as disciplinary strategies for disruptive behaviors resulting from OCD symptoms and otherwise. Please note that parents should always ensure that the child understands that the punishment is for the disruptive behavior and not the OCD symptom, ritual, or anxiety itself. Alternative responses (e.g., asking for more time rather than yelling) should be discussed with the child to ensure that she fully understands expectations and possible consequences.

Effective approach: rewarding

Rather than using punishment as a way to reduce OCD symptoms—discussed as an ineffective approach above—an alternative and more effective strategy is to provide rewards for attempts at ritual or compulsion reduction. Response prevention, or not allowing the compulsion to follow the obsession (see below for a discussion of exposure and response prevention, ERP), is one of the most effective techniques for reducing OCD symptoms. However, it can be difficult for children to engage in such actions, especially on their own, given the nature of OCD. Therefore, one way to increase compliance and decrease the interference of rituals, especially after a child has begun treatment and has an understanding of OCD and how obsessions and compulsions (as well as ERP) work, is to offer incentives for the child to push herself to confront anxious triggers without engaging in compulsions or rituals. For example, it may be helpful to set a timer for the child who experiences the ritual related to socks and shoes and to offer the incentive of using her iPad in the car on the way to school if she has her socks and shoes on by the time that the timer goes off. Use of if/then statements (e.g., "if you beat the buzzer with your socks, you may play on your iPad on the way to school," "if you touch the light switch only once on the way out of your room, you can pick the game we play downstairs," "if you eat from the plate prepared with no gloves, you can play outside after dinner for 30 minutes") can be very helpful in encouraging practice and effort in reducing compulsions despite feelings of anxiety.

Many parents think of rewards as bribes, but an important distinction is that bribes come before an action whereas rewards follow an action and are based on effort. Using rewards can be very effective and teach important lessons of effort and working for privileges while also giving good incentive to strive toward reducing OCD symptoms. There are many types of rewards. Traditionally items such as toys or food come to mind, but activity rewards, games, and privileges can be just as powerful if not more so. Varying rewards is important to ensure that the goal for the child's effort remains fresh and desirable.

Encouraging home practice

Cognitive behavioral therapy with exposure and response prevention (ERP)—either alone or together with medication in more severe presentations—is the most empirically supported form of treatment for OCD. However, most often, the successfulness of ERP depends on the amount of practice and exposure that the child is able to complete at home as well as the consistency with which the child (and family) is able to attend sessions and practice outside of session. Families should first seek care from a licensed mental health professional (MHP) who has training and experience in treatment of OCD using ERP. The professional will guide the child and parents in setting up a fear hierarchy, or a list of progressive activities to use for exposure/practice, and will begin demonstrating how to practice by having the child complete exposures in session. These activities will be easier at first and will become increasingly more difficult as the child gains more experience with practice and becomes more confident for "bossing back" the OCD symptoms. For example, if a child experiences rituals around germs, early exposures may be setting a timer for the amount of time she spends washing hands, or touching surfaces deemed as "mostly clean" (e.g., a desk, a toy), whereas later exposures may involve skipping hand washing altogether, especially if not absolutely necessary (reducing the number of times overall), or touching surfaces deemed as "dirty" (e.g., bathroom doorknob, floor). Once a child has conquered an activity in session with the MHP, she needs to practice at home in order to gain better confidence with the mastered step, further reduce anxiety, and generalize the newly found skill. The more that the child can practice at home, the better the outcome will be for treatment progression. However, it is also important to note that a child should not be pushed to practice beyond what has been prescribed in session by the MHP, unless the child feels that she is ready for the activity. Practices at home should feel manageable to the child and the parent, and should gradually increase in difficulty, mirroring exposures completed with the MHP in session.

Practice schedule

Many families have difficulty with consistent practice at home. Busy schedules, with multiple children, school, and extracurricular activities, not to mention possible resistance to practice (especially at first), can make completing exposures at home a difficult activity to conquer. Therefore, it can be helpful to set a schedule for home practice, in which for at least four days per week, a set time is carved into the daily family schedule to practice exposure for OCD symptoms.

There are two types of practice: planned practice and practice that occurs naturally. While natural exposures are also good for increasing gains, planned practices are likely going to provide the most benefit at home, at least during the first portion of treatment. Planned practices are more controlled and have set goals, which can be comforting to the child and parent. Setting a schedule for planned practices can help to maintain consistency at home and increase treatment benefits, while decreasing overall symptoms and the timeframe for treatment. When setting the schedule, it is important to allow enough time to complete the practice and for anxiety to decrease following the practice. It also may be helpful to plan a fun activity and/or reward following the practice, which the child may only participate in by complying with the exposure activity. For instance, for a child who is fearful of germs, and therefore has rituals about cleaning and re-cleaning dishes before eating or drinking, a planned practice may be drinking from three cups that are pulled from the cabinet (therefore the dishes have been previously washed and are clean) without washing or re-washing the cups prior to drinking. After the child has completed the activity, she may choose a game to play with the parent who is helping with the practice, or she may earn iPad time. The child should not be able to participate in the game or have iPad time until the planned exposure is complete. Once the child has completed several planned exposures of a similar nature (e.g., regarding dishes) and has gained confidence, the activity may be transitioned to occur more naturally. For example, an expectation may be set that dishes will not be re-washed prior to dinner each night. This rule should not be established until the child has mastered the activity in planned practice. As treatment progresses, planned practices will likely decrease in favor of natural practices for greater generalization of skills. However, families should do so with the guidance of their MHP.

The more practice the child completes, the greater confidence she will have for managing OCD symptoms and the less symptoms will interfere with daily life.

Resistance

Many children are resistant to practice, especially in the home setting where they feel most comfortable with pushing boundaries and have no outside influence or guidance. Parents take on a very important role during treatment by becoming the home coach when it is not possible for the MHP to be present. For this reason, parents should observe strategies used by the MHP to coax and encourage practice at a gradual pace. One such strategy is structure. Parents need to set a structure for how practices will be completed at home, with the understanding that participation is not optional. For instance, as described above, once the set time arrives, the child should understand exactly what is expected of him and should be asked to stay in the room with the parent until she chooses to engage in the practice activity. She should understand the potential reward that will follow the activity (e.g., you may play outside after you complete the practice) and that she will not be allowed to complete any other activities until practice time is over. Further, she should understand that disruptive behaviors are not acceptable during practice, and appropriate discipline strategies will be used if necessary.

Another important strategy is compromise. If a child indicates that a chosen practice exercise is too difficult, parents should work to find a compromise solution rather than abandon the practice altogether. For instance, the child may be asked to touch a dirty surface without washing and may resist. The parent could then suggest touching the surface instead of the child and have the child touch her hand. After the child has attempted the compromise, the parent may suggest trying the original activity again to earn the reward. To give another example, for a child who exhibits rituals for flipping the light switch three times, if only flipping the switch once is too hard, the child could be asked to flip the switch twice or flip the switch six times. Next, the parent could flip the switch once for the child prior to the child attempting to flip the switch once. In this way, the child continues to practice and get closer to the set goals, even if she feels that the original goal is too difficult. Children should be involved in suggesting compromises, as long as they can do so in a calm and realistic manner, as this will help them to engage in the practice activities and feel as if they are contributing to the process as well as being heard or understood.

With resistance, parents must use patience but also persistence. Acknowledging the difficulty of the task and the real experience of anxiety is important for the child, but it is also essential to understand and assert that practice is the method to decrease anxiety and is necessary for improvement. Most children will experience at least some resistance, especially at home in the environment in which they are most comfortable and experience the most compulsions. Therefore, having a plan for managing resistance prior to beginning practice exercises, or even practicing naturally, will assist in better management of anxiety and anxious oppositionality.

Maintaining gains

Learning to manage OCD symptoms is a journey for the child and her family. The journey takes time and will have good moments and tough moments. It is important to remember that once symptoms decrease or disappear altogether, the journey is not over. To maintain gains, children must continue to practice both actively and passively, and they must remember the skills they have learned to "boss back" their OCD. Parents are encouraged to schedule a regular check-in time at home at increasing intervals (once a week, once every two weeks, once a month) to discuss any new symptoms or any return of old symptoms that may have occurred and to help their child to make a plan to manage those symptoms if necessary. Parents and children should hold practices, especially for difficult tasks/challenging OCD symptoms, even after the family is no longer meeting with their MHP. Further, families may also wish to schedule one to two booster sessions with the MHP to ensure that everyone involved continues to practice learned skills to manage OCD symptoms. Booster sessions may be helpful as little as one month to six weeks after treatment completion or may not be needed until six months to a year following treatment, but there is no problem with returning for a refresher if needed. The MHP is there for support but should also encourage independence and continued growth. Based upon the CBT with ERP model, the same skills that are learned to combat one set of OCD symptoms (e.g., reducing washing for germ-related obsessions) can be applied for another set of OCD symptoms (e.g., reducing checking for safety-related obsessions). Therefore, once children and their parents learn how to manage OCD, those skills can be used as needed throughout life.

References

Chapter 1

Abramowitz, J.S., Fabricant, L.E., Taylor, S., Deacon, B.J., McKay, D., and Storch, E.A. (2014). The relevance of analogue studies for understanding obsessions and compulsions. *Clinical Psychology Review, 34*(3), 206–217.

Abramowitz, J.S., Taylor, S., and McKay, D. (2009). Obsessive-compulsive disorder. *The Lancet, 374*, 491–499.

APA (American Psychiatric Association) (2000). *Diagnostic and Statistical Manual of Mental Disorders* (4th edn, text revision). Washington, DC: APA.

APA (American Psychiatric Association) (2013). *Diagnostic and Statistical Manual of Mental Disorders* (5th edn). Arlington, VA: American Psychiatric Publishing.

Berman, N.C., Abramowitz, J.S., Pardue, C.M., and Wheaton, M.G. (2010). The relationship between religion and thought–action fusion: Use of an in vivo paradigm. *Behaviour Research and Therapy, 48*, 670–674.

Challis, C., Pelling, N., and Lack, C.W. (2008). The bio-psycho-social aspects and treatment of obsessive compulsive disorder: A primer for practitioners. *Australian Counseling Association Journal, 8*(1), 3–13.

De Mathis, M.A., Diniz, J.B., do Rosário, M.C., Torres, A.R. *et al.* (2006). What is the optimal way to subdivide obsessive-compulsive disorder? *CNS Spectrum, 11*(10), 762–768, 771–774, 776–779.

Fals-Stewart, W. and Angarano, K. (1994). Obsessive-compulsive disorder among patients entering substance abuse treatment: Prevalence and accuracy of diagnosis. *Journal of Nervous and Mental Disease, 182*(12), 715–719.

Fontenelle, I.S., Fontenelle, L.F., Borges, M.C., Prazeres *et al.* (2010). Quality of life and symptom dimensions of patients with obsessive-compulsive disorder. *Psychiatry Research, 179*(2), 198–203.

Fontenelle, L.F., Mendlowicz, M.V., Marques, C., and Versiani, M. (2004). Trans-cultural aspects of obsessive-compulsive disorder: A description of a Brazilian sample and a systematic review of international clinical studies. *Journal of Psychiatric Research, 38*, 403–411.

Franklin, M.E. and Foa, E.B. (2008). Obsessive-compulsive disorder. In D. Barlow (ed.), *Clinical Handbook of Psychological Disorders: A Step-by-Step Treatment Manual* (4th edn). New York: The Guilford Press.

Garcia-Soriano, G., Belloch, A., Morillo, C., and Clark, D.A. (2011). Symptom dimensions in obsessive–compulsive disorder: From normal cognitive intrusions to clinical obsessions. *Journal of Anxiety Disorders, 25*, 474–482.

Geller, D. (2006). Obsessive-compulsive and spectrum disorders in children and adolescents. *Psychiatric Clinics of North America, 29,* 353–370.

Geller, D.A., Biederman, J., Griffin, S., Jones, J., and Lefkowitz, T.R. (1996) Comorbidity of juvenile obsessive-compulsive disorder with disruptive behavior disorders. *Journal of the American Academy of Child & Adolescent Psychiatry, 35*(12), 1637–1646.

Kanner, A.M. (2005). Depression in epilepsy: A neurobiologic perspective. *Epilepsy Currents, 5*(1), 21–27. doi:10.1111/j.1535-7597.2005.05106.x

Kessler R., Berglund, P., Demler, O., Jin, R., and Walters, E. (2005). Lifetime prevalence and age-of-onset distributions of DSM-IV disorders in the National Comorbidity Survey Replication. *Archives of General Psychiatry, 62*, 593–602.

Krochmalik, A. and Menzies, R. (2003). The classification and diagnosis of obsessive–compulsive disorder. In R.G. Menzies and P. de Silva (eds), *Obsessive–Compulsive Disorder: Theory, Research, and Treatment*. New York: Wiley.

Lack, C.W. (2013). *Anxiety Disorders: An Introduction*. Fareham, UK: Onus Books.

Lack, C.W., Huskey, A., Weed, D.B., Highfill, M.J., and Craig, L. (2015). The etiology of obsessive-compulsive disorder. In C.W. Lack (ed.), *Obsessive-Compulsive Disorder: Etiology, Phenomenology, and Treatment*. Fareham, UK: Onus Books.

Lack, C.W., Storch, E.A., Keeley, M.L., Geffken, G.R., Ricketts, E.D., Murphy, T.K., and Goodman, W.K. (2009). Quality of life in children and adolescents with obsessive–compulsive disorder: Base rates, parent–child agreement, and clinical correlates. *Social Psychiatry and Psychiatric Epidemiology, 44*(11), 935–942.

Leckman, J.F., Denys, D., Simpson, H.B., Mataix-Cols, D. *et al.* (2010). Obsessive-compulsive disorder: A review of the diagnostic criteria and possible subtypes and dimensional specifiers for DSM-5. *Depression and Anxiety, 27*, 507–527.

Macy, A.S., Theo, J.N., Kaufmann, S.C., Chazzaoui, R.B. *et al.* (2013). Quality of life in obsessive compulsive disorder. *CNS Spectrum, 18*(1), 21–33.

Piacentini, J., Peris, T.S., Bergman, R.L., Chang, S., and Jaffer, M. (2007). Functional impairment in childhood OCD: development and psychometrics properties of the child obsessive-compulsive impact scale-revised (COIS-R). *Journal of Clinical Child and Adolescent Psychology, 36,* 645–653.

Ruscio, A.M., Stein, D.J., Chiu, W.T., and Kessler, R.C. (2010). The epidemiology of obsessive-compulsive disorder in the National Comorbidity Survey Replication. *Molecular Psychiatry, 15,* 53–63.

Salzman, L. and Thaler, F. (1981). Obsessive-compulsive disorders: A review of the literature. *American Journal of Psychiatry, 138,* 286–296.

Stein, D.J., Fineberg, N.A., Bienvenu, O.J., Denys, D. *et al.* (2010). Should OCD be classified as an anxiety disorder in *DSM-5*? *Depression and Anxiety, 27,* 495–506.

Stewart, S.E., Rosario, M.C., Baer, L., Carter, A.S. *et al.* (2008). Four-factor structure of obsessive-compulsive disorder symptoms in children, adolescents, and adults. *Journal of the American Academy of Child & Adolescent Psychiatry, 47*(7), 763–772.

Storch, E.A., Abramowitz, J., and Goodman, W.K. (2008). Where does obsessive-compulsive disorder belong in the DSM-V? *Depression and Anxiety, 25*(4), 336–347.

Subramaniam, M., Soh, P., Vaingankar, J.A., Picco, L., and Chong, S.A. (2013). Quality of life in obsessive–compulsive disorder: Impact of the disorder and of treatment. *CNS Drugs, 27*(5), 367–383.

Torres, A., Prince, M., Bebbington, P., Psych, M.R.C. *et al.* (2006). Obsessive-compulsive disorder: Prevalence, comorbidity, impact, and help-seeking in the British National Psychiatric Comorbidity Survey of 2000. *The American Journal of Psychiatry, 163*(11), 1978–1985.

WHO (World Health Organization) (2010) *International Statistical Classification of Diseases and Related Health Problems 10th Revision (ICD-10)* (4th edn). Available at: www.who.int/classifications/icd/en/bluebook. pdf, accessed on 24 October 2016.

Williams, M.T. and Steever, A. (2015). Cultural manifestations of obsessive-compulsive disorder. In C.W. Lack (ed.), *Obsessive-Compulsive Disorder: Etiology, Phenomenology, and Treatment.* Fareham, UK: Onus Books.

Zohar, A.H. (1999). The epidemiology of obsessive-compulsive disorder in children and adolescents. *Child and Adolescent Psychiatric Clinics of North America, 8,* 445–460.

Chapter 3

Abramovitch, A., Abramowitz, J.S., Mittleman, A., Stark, A., Ramsey, K., and Geller, D.A. (2015). Neuropsychological test performance in pediatric obsessive-compulsive disorder: A meta-analysis. *Journal of Child Psychology & Psychiatry, 56*(8), 837–847.

Abramovitch, A. and Cooperman, A. (2015). The cognitive neuropsychology of obsessive-compulsive disorder: A critical review. *Journal of Obsessive-Compulsive and Related Disorders, 5*(1), 24–36.

Abramowitz, J.S., Franklin, M.E., Schwartz, S.A., and Furr, J.M. (2003). Symptom presentation and outcome of cognitive-behavioral therapy for obsessive-compulsive disorder. *Journal of Consulting and Clinical Psychology, 71*(6), 1049–1057.

Abramowitz, J.S., Taylor, S., and McKay, D. (2009). Obsessive-compulsive disorder. *Lancet, 374,* 489–497.

Albert, P.R., Benkelfat, C., and Descarries, L. (2012). The neurobiology of depression: Revisiting the serotonin hypothesis. I. Cellular and molecular mechanisms. *Philosophical Transactions of the Royal Society of London: Series B, Biological Sciences, 367*(1601), 2378–2381.

Alvarenga, P.G., Cesar, R.C., Leckman, J.F., Moriyama, T.S. *et al.* (2015). Obsessive compulsive symptom dimensions in a population-based, cross-sectional sample of school-aged children. *Journal of Psychiatric Research, 62,* 108–114.

APA (American Psychiatric Association) (2013). *Diagnostic and Statistical Manual of Mental Disorders* (5th edn). Arlington, VA: American Psychiatric Publishing.

Black, D.W., Stumpf, A., McCormick, B., Allen, J., Blum, N., and Noyes, R. (2013). A blind re-analysis of the Iowa family study of obsessive-compulsive disorder. *Psychiatry Research, 209*(2), 202–206.

Browne, H.A., Gair, S.L., Scharf, J.M., and Grice, D.E. (2014). Genetics of obsessive-compulsive disorder and related disorders. *Psychiatric Clinics of North America, 37*(3), 319–335.

Browne, H.A., Hansen, S.N., Buxbaum, J.D., Gair, S.L. *et al.* (2015). Familial clustering of tic disorders and obsessive-compulsive disorder. *JAMA Psychiatry, 72*(4), 359–366.

Byrne, S.P., Rapee, R.M., Richardson, R., Malhi, G.S., Jones, M., and Hudson, J.L. (2015). D-cycloserine enhances generalization of fear extinction in children. *Depress and Anxiety, 32*(6), 408–414.

Craske, M.G. (2003). *Origins of Phobias and Anxiety Disorders: Why More Women Than Men?* Amsterdam: Elsevier.

Craske, M.G., Treanor, M., Conway, C.C., Zbozinek, T., and Vervliet, B. (2014). Maximizing exposure therapy: An inhibitory learning approach. *Behaviour Research and Therapy, 58,* 10–23.

Eisen, J.L., Sibrava, N.J., Boisseau, C.L., Mancebo, M.C. *et al.* (2013). Five-year course of obsessive-compulsive disorder: Predictors of remission and relapse. *Journal of Clinical Psychiatry, 74*(3), 233–239.

Foa, E.B. and Kozak, M.J. (1986). Emotional processing of fear: Exposure to corrective information. *Psychological Bulletin, 99*(1), 20–35.

Franklin, M.E., Kratz, H.E., Freeman, J.B., Ivarsson, T. (2015). Cognitive-behavioral therapy for pediatric obsessive-compulsive disorder: Empirical review and clinical recommendations. *Psychiatry Research, 227*(1), 78–92.

Freud, S. (1895). Obsessions and phobias: Their physical mechanisms and their etiology. *Standard Edition, 1,* 70–84.

Greisberg, S. and McKay, D. (2003). Neuropsychology of obsessive-compulsive disorder: A review and treatment implications. *Clinical Psychology Review, 23*(1), 95–117.

Gross, R., Sasson, Y., Chopra, M., and Zohar, J. (1998). Biological models of obsessive-compulsive disorder: the serotonin hypothesis. In R.P. Swinson, M. Antony, S. Rachman, and M.A. Richter (eds), *Obsessive-Compulsive Disorder: Theory, Research, and Treatment.* New York: The Guilford Press.

Harkin, B. and Kessler, K. (2011). The role of working memory in compulsive checking and OCD: A systematic classification of 58 experimental findings. *Clinical Psychology Review, 31,* 1004–1021.

Hollon, S.D., Arean, P.A., Craske, M.G., Crawford, K.A. *et al.* (2014). Development of clinical practice guidelines. *Annual Review of Clinical Psychology, 10,* 213–241.

Insel, T., Cuthbert, B., Garvey, M., Heinssen, R. *et al.* (2010). Research Domain Criteria (RDoC): Toward a new classification framework for research on mental disorders. *American Journal of Psychiatry, 167*(7), 748–751.

Ivarsson, T., Skarphedinsson, G., Kornor, H., Axelsdottir, B. *et al.* (2015). The place of and evidence for serotonin reuptake inhibitors (SRIs) for obsessive compulsive disorder (OCD) in children and adolescents: Views based on a systematic review and meta-analysis. *Psychiatry Research, 227*(1), 93–103.

Janet, P. (1903). Les obsessions et la psychasthénie. (2nd edn, M.W. Adamowicz, trans.). Paris: Alcan.

Keeley, M.L., Storch, E.A., Merlo, L.J., and Geffken, G.R. (2008). Clinical predictors of response to cognitive-behavioral therapy for obsessive-compulsive disorder. *Clinical Psychology Review, 28*(1), 118–130.

Kendler, K.S. (2005). "A Gene for...": The nature of gene action in psychiatric disorders. *American Journal of Psychiatry, 162,* 1243–1252.

Kichuk, S.A., Torres, A.R., Fontenelle, L.F., Rosario, M.C. *et al.* (2013). Symptom dimensions are associated with age of onset and clinical course of obsessive-compulsive disorder. *Progress in Neuro-Psychopharmacology and Biological Psychiatry, 44,* 233–239.

Kim, S.K., McKay, D., Taylor, S., Tolin, D. *et al.* (2016). The structure of obsessive compulsive symptoms and beliefs: A correspondence and biplot analysis. *Journal of Anxiety Disorders, 38,* 79–87.

Kringlen, E. (1965). Obsessional neurotics: Long-term outcome. *British Journal of Psychiatry, 111,* 709–722.

Lebowitz, E.R., Scharfstein, L.A., and Jones, J. (2014). Comparing family accommodation in pediatric obsessive-compulsive disorder, anxiety disorders, and nonanxious children. *Depression and Anxiety, 31*(12), 1018–1025.

Ludvik, D., Boschen, M.J., and Neuman, D.L. (2015). Effective behavioural strategies for reducing disgust in contamination-related OCD: A review. *Clinical Psychology Review, 42,* 116–129.

Markarian, Y., Larson, M.J., Aldea, M.A., Baldwin, S.A. *et al.* (2010). Multiple pathways to functional impairment in obsessive-compulsive disorder. *Clinical Psychology Review, 30*(1), 78–88.

Mason, E.C. and Richardson, R. (2012). Treating disgust in anxiety disorders. *Clinical Psychology: Science and Practice, 19*(2), 180–194.

Mataix-Cols, D., Boman, M., Monzani, B., Ruck, C. *et al.* (2013). Population-based, multigenerational family clustering study of obsessive-compulsive disorder. *JAMA Psychiatry, 70*(7), 709–717.

McCain, J.A. (2009). Antidepressants and suicide in adolescents and adults. *Pharmacy and Therapeutics, 34*(7), 355–367.

McGuire, J.F., Crawford, E.A., Park, J.M., Storch, E.A. *et al.* (2014). Neuropsychological performance across symptom dimensions in pediatric obsessive compulsive disorder. *Depression and Anxiety, 31,* 988–996.

McGuire, J.F., Orr, S.P., Wu, M.S., Lewin, A.B. *et al.* (2016). Fear conditioning and extinction in youth with obsessive-compulsive disorder. *Depression and Anxiety, 33*(3), 229–237.

McKay, D. (2006). Treating disgust reactions in contamination-based obsessive-compulsive disorder. *Journal of Behavioral Therapy and Experimental Psychiatry, 37*(1), 53–59.

McKay, D. and Tolin, D.F. (2016). Empirically supported psychological treatments and the research domain criteria (RDoC). under review.

McKay, D., Piacentini, J., Greisberg, S., Graae, F., Jaffer, M., and Miller, J. (2006). The structure of childhood obsessions and compulsions: Dimensions in an outpatient sample. *Behaviour Research and Therapy, 44*(1), 137–146.

McKay, D., Sookman, D., Neziroglu, F., Wilhelm, S. *et al.* (2015). Efficacy of cognitive-behavioral therapy for obsessive-compulsive disorder. *Psychiatry Research, 225*(3), 236–246.

Nissen, J.B., Nikolajsen, K.H., and Thomsen, P.H. (2014). A 7-year follow-up of children and adolescents with obsessive-compulsive disorder: An analysis of predictive factors in a clinical prospective study. *European Journal of Psychiatry, 28*(3), 183–193.

Olatunji, B.O. and McKay, D. (2007). Disgust and psychiatric illness: Have we remembered? *The British Journal of Psychiatry, 190,* 457–459.

Piras, F., Piras, F., Chiapponi, C., Girardi, P., Caltagirone, C., and Spalletta, G. (2015). Widespread structural brain changes in OCD: A systematic review of voxel-based morphometry studies. *Cortex, 62,* 89–108.

Salkovskis, P. (1985). Obsessional–compulsive problems: A cognitive-behavioural analysis. *Behaviour Research and Therapy, 23*(5), 571–583.

Samuels, J. and Nestadt, G. (1997). Epidemiology and genetics of obsessive-compulsive disorder. *International Review of Psychiatry, 9*(1), 61–72.

Sharma, E., Thennarasu, K., and Reddy, Y.C.J. (2014). Long-term outcome of obsessive–compulsive disorder in adults: A meta-analysis. *Journal of Clinical Psychiatry, 75*(9), 1019–1027.

Snider, L.A. and Swedo, S.E. (2000). Pediatric obsessive-compulsive disorder. *JAMA, 284*(24), 3104–3106.

Snyder, H.R., Kaiser, R.H., Warren, S.L., and Heller, W. (2015). Obsessive-compulsive disorder is associated with broad impairments in executive function: A meta-analysis. *Clinical Psychological Science, 3*(2), 301–330.

Stewart, S.E., Yu, D., Scharf, J.M., Neale, B.M. *et al.* (2013). Genome-wide association study of obsessive compulsive disorder. *Molecular Psychiatry, 18,* 788–798.

Taylor, S. (2013). Molecular genetics of obsessive-compulsive disorder: A comprehensive meta-analysis of genetic association studies. *Molecular Psychiatry, 18,* 799–805.

Taylor, S., Abramowitz, J.S., McKay, D., Calamari, J.E. *et al.* (2006). Do dysfunctional beliefs play a role in all types of obsessive-compulsive disorder? *Journal of Anxiety Disorders, 20*(1), 85–97.

Thorsen, A.L., van den Heuvel, O., and Hansen, B. (2015). Neuroimaging of psychotherapy for obsessive-compulsive disorder: A systematic review. *Psychiatry Research: Neuroimaging, 233*(3), 306–313.

Tolin, D.F., McKay, D., Forman, E.M., Klonsky, E.D., and Thombs, B.D. (2015). Empirically supported treatment: Recommendations for a new model. *Clinical Psychology: Science and Practice, 22*(4), 317–338.

Tolin, D.F., Worhunsky, P., and Maltby, N. (2006). Are "obsessive" beliefs specific to OCD?: A comparison across anxiety disorders. *Behaviour Research and Therapy, 44*(4), 469–480.

Torresan, R.C., Ramos-Cerqueira, A.T.A., Shavitt, R.G., do Rosario, M.C. *et al.* (2013). Symptom dimensions, clinical course and comorbidity in men and women with obsessive-compulsive disorder. *Psychiatry Research, 209*(2), 186–195.

Yarbro, J., Mahaffey, B., Abramowitz, J., and Kashdan, T.B. (2013). Recollections of parent-child relationships, attachment insecurity, and obsessive-compulsive beliefs. *Personality and Individual Differences, 54*(3), 355–360.

Yaryura-Tobias, J., Grunes, M.S., Todaro, J., McKay, D., Neziroglu, F.A., and Stockman, R. (2000). Nosological insertion of Axis I disorders in the etiology of obsessive-compulsive disorder. *Journal of Anxiety Disorders, 14*(1), 19–30.

Zohar, A.H. (1999). The epidemiology of obsessive-compulsive disorder in children and adolescents. *Child and Adolescent Psychiatric Clinics of North America, 8*(3), 445–460.

Chapter 4

APA (American Psychiatric Association) (2013). *Diagnostic and Statistical Manual of Mental Disorders* (5th edn). Arlington, VA: American Psychiatric Publishing.

Brown, T.A., Moras, K., Zinbarg, R.E., and Barlow, D.H. (1993). Diagnostic and symptom distinguishability of generalized anxiety disorder and obsessive-compulsive disorder. *Behavior Therapy, 24*, 227–240.

Chapter 5

Bloch, M.H. and Storch, E.A. (2015). Assessment and management of treatment-refractory obsessive-compulsive disorder in children. *Journal of the American Academy of Child & Adolescent Psychiatry, 54*, 251–262.

Franklin, M.E., Kratz, H.E., Freeman, J.B., Ivarsson, T. *et al.* (2015). Cognitive-behavioral therapy for pediatric obsessive-compulsive disorder: Empirical review and clinical recommendations. *Psychiatry Research, 227*, 78–92.

Geller, D.A., Biederman, J., Stewart, S.E., Mullin, B. *et al.* (2003a). Impact of comorbidity on treatment response to paroxetine in pediatric obsessive-compulsive disorder: Is the use of exclusion criteria empirically supported in randomized clinical trials? *Journal of Child and Adolescent Psychopharmacology, 13*, 19–29.

Geller, D.A., Biederman, J., Stewart, S.E., Mullin, B. *et al.* (2003b). Which SSRI? A meta-analysis of pharmacotherapy trials in pediatric obsessive-compulsive disorder. *American Journal of Psychiatry, 160,* 1919–1928.

Geller, D.A. and March, J. (2012). Practice parameter for the assessment and treatment of children and adolescents with obsessive-compulsive disorder. *Journal of the American Academy of Child & Adolescent Psychiatry, 51,* 98–113.

Lewin, A.B., McGuire, J.F., Murphy, T.K., and Storch, E.A. (2014). Editorial perspective: The importance of considering parent's preferences when planning treatment for their children—the case of childhood obsessive-compulsive disorder. *Journal of Child Psychology and Psychiatry, 55,* 1314–1316.

POTS (Pediatric OCD Treatment Study) (2004). Cognitive-behavior therapy, sertraline, and their combination for children and adolescents with obsessive-compulsive disorder: The Pediatric OCD Treatment Study (POTS) randomized controlled trial. *JAMA, 292,* 1969–1976.

March, J.S., Franklin, M.E., Leonard, H., Garcia, A. *et al.* (2007). Tics moderate treatment outcome with sertraline but not cognitive-behavior therapy in pediatric obsessive-compulsive disorder. *Biological Psychiatry, 61,* 344–347.

McGuire, J.F., Piacentini, J., Lewin, A.B., Brennan, E.A., Murphy, T.K., and Storch, E.A. (2015). A meta-analysis of cognitive behavior therapy and medication for child obsessive compulsive disorder: Moderators of treatment efficacy, response, and remission. *Depression & Anxiety 32*(8), 580–593.

O'Leary, E.M.M., Barrett, P., and Fjermestad, K.W. (2009). Cognitive-behavioral family treatment for childhood obsessive-compulsive disorder: A 7-year follow-up study. *Journal of Anxiety Disorders, 23,* 973–978.

Scahill, L., Riddle, M.A., McSwiggin-Hardin, M., Ort, S.I. *et al.* (1997). Children's Yale-Brown obsessive compulsive scale: Reliability and validity. *Journal of the American Academy of Child & Adolescent Psychiatry, 36,* 844–852.

Skarphedinsson, G., Weidle, B., Thomsen, P.H., Dahl, K. *et al.* (2015). Continued cognitive-behavior therapy versus sertraline for children and adolescents with obsessive–compulsive disorder that were non-responders to cognitive-behavior therapy: A randomized controlled trial. *European Child & Adolescent Psychiatry, 24*(5), 591–602.

Storch, E.A., Bussing, R., Small, B.J., Geffken, G.R. *et al.* (2013). Randomized, placebo-controlled trial of cognitive-behavioral therapy alone or combined with sertraline in the treatment of pediatric obsessive–compulsive disorder. *Behaviour Research and Therapy, 51,* 823–829.

Chapter 6

Bell, J. (2007). *Rewind, Replay, Repeat: A Memoir of Obsessive-Compulsive Disorder*. Center City, MN: Hazelden Publishing.

Ivarsson, T., Skarphedinsson, G., Kornor, H., Axelsdottir, B. *et al.* (2015). The place of and evidence for serotonin reuptake inhibitors (SRIs) for obsessive compulsive disorder (OCD) in children and adolescents: Views based on a systematic review and meta-analysis. *Psychiatry Research, 227*(1), 93–103.

March, J.S. and Mulle, K. (1998). *OCD in Children and Adolescents: A Cognitive-Behavioral Treatment Manual*. New York: The Guilford Press.

McGuire, J.F., Piacentini, J., Lewin, A.B., Brennan, E.A., Murphy, T.K., and Storch, E.A. (2015). A meta-analysis of cognitive-behavioral therapy and medication for child obsessive-compulsive disorder: Moderators of treatment efficacy, response, and remission. *Depression and Anxiety, 32*, 580–593.

Chapter 8

APA (American Psychological Association) (1995). Division of Clinical Psychology, Task Force on Promotion and Dissemination of Psychological Procedures. Training in and dissemination of empirically-validated psychological treatments: Report on recommendations. *Clinical Psychologist, 48*, 3–23.

Barrett, P., Farrell, L., Dadds, M., and Boulter, N. (2005). Cognitive-behavioral family treatment of childhood obsessive-compulsive disorder: Long-term follow-up and predictors of outcome. *Journal of the American Academy of Child & Adolescent Psychiatry, 44*, 1005–1014.

Berlin, H.A., Koran, L.M., Jenike, M.A., Shapira, N.A., *et al.* (2011). Double-blind, placebo-controlled trial of topiramate augmentation in treatment-resistant obsessive-compulsive disorder. *Journal of Clinical Psychiatry, 72*, 716.

Bipeta, R., Yerramilli, S.S., Pingali, S., Karredla, A.R., and Ali, M.O. (2013). A cross-sectional study of insight and family accommodation in pediatric obsessive-compulsive disorder. *Child and Adolescent Psychiatry and Mental Health, 7*, 20.

Bloch, M.H., Landeros-Weisenberger, A., Kelmendi, B., Coric, V., *et al.* (2006). A systematic review: Antipsychotic augmentation with treatment refractory obsessive-compulsive disorder. *Molecular Psychiatry, 11*(7), 622–632.

Bloch, M.H. and Storch, E.A. (2015). Assessment and management of treatment-refractory obsessive-compulsive disorder in children. *Journal of the American Academy of Child & Adolescent Psychiatry, 54*, 251–262.

Chu, B.C., Colognori, D.B., Yang, G., Xie, M.G., Bergman, R.L., and Piacentini, J. (2015). Mediators of exposure therapy for youth obsessive-compulsive disorder: Specificity and temporal sequence of client and treatment factors. *Behavior Therapy, 46*, 395–408.

Coric, V., Taskiran, S., Pittenger, C., Wasylink, S., *et al.* (2005). Riluzole augmentation in treatment-resistant obsessive–compulsive disorder: An open-label trial. *Biological Psychiatry, 58*, 424–428.

Diniz, J.B., Shavitt, R.G., Pereira, C.A.B., Hounie, A.G., *et al.* (2010). Quetiapine versus clomipramine in the augmentation of selective serotonin reuptake inhibitors for the treatment of obsessive-compulsive disorder: A randomized, open-label trial. *Journal of Psychopharmacology, 24*, 297–307.

Franklin, M.E., Sapyta, J., Freeman, J. B., Khanna, M., *et al.* (2011). Cognitive behavior therapy augmentation of pharmacotherapy in pediatric obsessive-compulsive disorder: The Pediatric OCD Treatment Study II (POTS II) randomized controlled trial. *JAMA, 306*, 1224–1232.

Geller, D.A., Biederman, J., Stewart, S.E., *et al.* (2003). Which SSRI? A meta-analysis of pharmacotherapy trials in pediatric obsessive-compulsive disorder. *American Journal of Psychiatry, 11*, 1919–1928.

Geller, D.A., and March, J. (2012). Practice parameter for the assessment and treatment of children and adolescents with obsessive-compulsive disorder. *Focus, 10*, 360–373.

Goodman, W.K., Price, L.H., Rasmussen, S.A., Mazure, C., *et al.* (1989). The Yale-Brown obsessive compulsive scale: I. Development, use, and reliability. *Archives of General Psychiatry, 46*, 1006–1011.

Grant, P.J., Joseph, L.A., Farmer, C.A., Luckenbaugh, D.A., *et al.* (2014). 12-week, placebo-controlled trial of add-on riluzole in the treatment of childhood-onset obsessive–compulsive disorder. *Neuropsychopharmacology, 39*, 1453–1459.

Grant, P., Lougee, L., Hirschtritt, M., and Swedo, S.E. (2007). An open-label trial of riluzole, a glutamate antagonist, in children with treatment-resistant obsessive-compulsive disorder. *Journal of Child and Adolescent Psychopharmacology, 17*, 761–767.

Guy, W. (1976). *Clinical Global Impression Scale: The ECDEU Assessment Manual for Psychopharmacology*, revised. Rockville, MD: National Institute of Mental Health.

Jordan, C., Reid, A.M., Mariaskin, A., Augusto, B., and Sulkowski, M.L. (2012). First-line treatment for pediatric obsessive–compulsive disorder. *Journal of Contemporary Psychotherapy, 42*, 243–248.

Kariuki-Nyuthe, C., Gomez-Mancilla, B., and Stein, D.J. (2014). Obsessive compulsive disorder and the glutamatergic system. *Current Opinion in Psychiatry, 27*, 32–37.

Lewin, A.B., Bergman, R.L., Peris, T.S., Chang, S., McCracken, J.T., and Piacentini, J. (2010). Correlates of insight among youth with obsessive-compulsive disorder. *Journal of Child Psychology and Psychiatry, 51*, 603–611.

Maltby, N. and Tolin, D.F. (2005). A brief motivational intervention for treatment-refusing OCD patients. *Cognitive Behaviour Therapy, 34*, 176–184.

McElroy, S.L., Arnold, L.M., Shapira, N.A., Keck Jr, P.E., *et al.* (2014). Topiramate in the treatment of binge eating disorder associated with obesity: A randomized, placebo-controlled trial. *American Journal of Psychiatry, 2*, 255–261.

Merlo, L.J., Storch, E.A., Lehmkuhl, H.D., Jacob, M.L., *et al.* (2010). Cognitive behavioral therapy plus motivational interviewing improves outcome for pediatric obsessive–compulsive disorder: A preliminary study. *Cognitive Behaviour Therapy, 39*, 24–27.

Miller, W., Rollnick, S., and Conforti, K. (2002). *Motivational Interviewing: Preparing People for Change (2nd edn)*. New York: The Guilford Press.

Mowla, A., Khajeian, A.M., Sahraian, A., Chohedri, A.H., and Kashkoli, F. (2010). Topiramate augmentation in resistant OCD: A double-blind placebo-controlled clinical trial. *CNS Spectrums, 15*, 613–617.

Pallanti, S., Hollander, E., Bienstock, C., Koran, L., *et al.* (2002). Treatment non-response in OCD: Methodological issues and operational definitions. *International Journal of Neuropsychopharmacology, 5*, 181–191.

Pallanti, S., Quercioli, L., Paiva, R.S., and Koran, L.M. (1999). Citalopram for treatment-resistant obsessive-compulsive disorder. *European Psychiatry, 14*, 101–106.

Pence Jr, S.L., Sulkowski, M.L., Jordan, C., and Storch, E.A. (2010). When exposures go wrong: Trouble-shooting guidelines for managing difficult scenarios that arise in exposure-based treatment for obsessive-compulsive disorder. *American Journal of Psychotherapy, 64*, 39–53.

Pittenger, C., Kelmendi, B., Wasylink, S., Bloch, M.H., and Coric, V. (2008). Riluzole augmentation in treatment-refractory obsessive-compulsive disorder: A series of 13 cases, with long-term follow-up. *Journal of Clinical Psychopharmacology, 28*, 363–367.

POTS (Pediatric OCD Treatment Study Team) (2004). Cognitive-behavior therapy, sertraline, and their combination with children and adolescents with Obsessive-Compulsive Disorder: The Pediatric OCD Treatment Study (POTS) randomized controlled trial. *JAMA, 292*, 1969–1976.

Rahman, O., Ale, C., Sulkowski, M.L., and Storch, E.A. (2013). Treatment of comorbid anxiety and disruptive behavior. In E.A. Storch and D. McKay (eds), *Handbook of Treating Variants and Complications in Anxiety Disorders*. New York, NY: Springer.

Simpson, H.B., Foa, E.B., Liebowitz, M.R., Huppert, J.D., *et al.* (2013). Cognitive-behavioral therapy vs risperidone for augmenting serotonin reuptake inhibitors in obsessive-compulsive disorder: A randomized clinical trial. *JAMA Psychiatry, 70,* 1190–1199.

Storch, E.A., De Nadai, A.S., Jacob, M.L., Lewin, A.B., *et al.* (2014). Phenomenology and correlates of insight in pediatric obsessive–compulsive disorder. *Comprehensive Psychiatry, 55,* 613–620.

Storch, E.A., Geffken, G.R., Merlo, L.J., Jacob, M.L., *et al.* (2007). Family accommodation in pediatric obsessive–compulsive disorder. *Journal of Clinical Child and Adolescent Psychology, 36,* 207–216.

Storch, E.A., Jones, A.M., Lack, C.W., Ale, C.M., *et al.* (2012). Rage attacks in pediatric obsessive-compulsive disorder: Phenomenology and clinical correlates. *Journal of the American Academy of Child & Adolescent Psychiatry, 51,* 582–592.

Storch, E.A., Lehmkuhl, H.D., Ricketts, E., Geffken, G.R., Marien, W., and Murphy, T.K. (2010). An open trial of intensive family based cognitive-behavioral therapy in youth with obsessive-compulsive disorder who are medication partial responders or nonresponders. *Journal of Clinical Child & Adolescent Psychology, 39,* 260–268.

Storch, E.A., Merlo, L.J., Larson, M.J., Geffken, G.R., *et al.* (2008). Impact of comorbidity on cognitive-behavioral therapy response in pediatric obsessive-compulsive disorder. *Journal of the American Academy of Child & Adolescent Psychiatry, 47,* 583–592.

Sulkowski, M.L., Geller, D.A., Lewin, A.B., Murphy, T.K., *et al.* (2014). The future of d-cycloserine and other cognitive modifiers in obsessive-compulsive and related disorders. *Current Psychiatry Reviews, 10,* 317–324.

Watson, H.J. and Rees, C.S. (2008). Meta-analysis of randomized, controlled treatment trials for pediatric obsessive-compulsive disorder. *Journal of Child Psychology and Psychiatry, 49,* 489–498.

Chapter 10

Barrett, P., Farrell, L., Dadds, M., and Boulter, N. (2005). Cognitive-behavioral family treatment of childhood obsessive-compulsive disorder: Long-term follow-up and predictors of outcome. *Journal of the American Academy of Child & Adolescent Psychiatry, 44,* 1005–1014.

Comer, J.S., Furr, J.M., Cooper-Vince, C.E., Kerns, C.E., *et al.* (2014). Internet-delivered, family-based treatment for early-onset OCD: A preliminary case series. *Journal of Clinical Child & Adolescent Psychology, 43,* 74–87.

Freeman, J., Garcia, A., Frank, H., Benito, K., *et al.* (2014). Evidence base update for psychosocial treatments for pediatric obsessive-compulsive disorder. *Journal of Clinical Child & Adolescent Psychology, 43,* 7–26.

Jaurrieta, N., Jimenez-Murcia, S., Alonso, P., Granero, R., *et al.* (2008). Individual versus group cognitive behavioral treatment for obsessive-compulsive disorder: Follow up. *Psychiatry and Clinical Neurosciences, 62,* 697–704.

Jonsson, H. and Hougaard, E. (2009). Group cognitive behavioural therapy for obsessive-compulsive disorder: A systematic review and meta-analysis. *Acta Psychiatrica Scandinavica, 119,* 98–106.

Lewin, A.B., McGuire, J.F., Murphy, T.K., and Storch, E.A. (2014). Editorial perspective: The importance of considering parents' preferences when planning treatment for their children—The case of childhood obsessive-compulsive disorder. *Journal of Child Psychology and Psychiatry, 55*(12), 1314–1316.

Lewin, A.B., Storch, E.A., Adkins, J., Murphy, T.K., and Geffken, G.R. (2005a). Current directions in pediatric obsessive-compulsive disorder. *Pediatric Annals, 34*(2), 128–134.

Lewin, A.B., Storch, E.A., Merlo, L.J., Adkins, J.W., Murphy, T.K., and Geffken, G.R. (2005b). Intensive cognitive behavioral therapy for pediatric obsessive-compulsive disorder: A treatment protocol for mental health providers. *Psychological Services, 2,* 91–104.

POTS (Pediatric OCD Treatment Study) (2004). Cognitive-behavior therapy, sertraline, and their combination for children and adolescents with obsessive-compulsive disorder: The Pediatric OCD Treatment Study (POTS) randomized controlled trial. *JAMA, 292,* 1969–1976.

Storch, E.A., Caporino, N.E., Morgan, J.R., Lewin, A.B., *et al.* (2011). Preliminary investigation of web-camera delivered cognitive-behavioral therapy for youth with obsessive-compulsive disorder. *Psychiatry Research, 189,* 407–412.

Turner, C.M., Mataix-Cols, D., Lovell, K., Krebs, G., et al. (2014). Telephone cognitive-behavioral therapy for adolescents with obsessive-compulsive disorder: A randomized controlled non-inferiority trial. *Journal of the American Academy of Child & Adolescent Psychiatry, 53,* 1298–1307.

Chapter 11

Leininger, M., Dyches, T.T., Prater, M.A., and Heath, M.A. (2010). Teaching students with obsessive-compulsive disorder. *Intervention in School and Clinic, 45,* 221–231.

Storch, E.A. and Merlo, L.J. (2006). Obsessive-compulsive disorder: Strategies for using CBT and pharmacotherapy. *Journal of Family Practice,* 55(4), 329–334.

Subject Index

Author Index